Mentoring in N

About the Author

Sheila C. Grossman, PhD, APRN-BC, received her baccalaureate and doctoral degrees from the University of Connecticut, her master's degree from the University of Massachusetts in biophysiological nursing with a clinical nurse specialty in respiratory nursing, and her post-master's certificate as a family nurse practitioner from Fairfield University. Grossman has completed the Cincinnati Children's Hospital Genetics Fellowship and the AACN Leadership Fellowship. She has practiced as a staff and charge nurse on a variety of medical-surgical and critical care units and has been a critical care instructor at Hartford Hospital and St. Francis Hospital and Medical Center in Hartford, Connecticut. She has taught nursing at the University of Connecticut and currently is a professor and specialty director of the Family Nurse Practitioner Program at Fairfield University, Fairfield, Connecticut, and affiliates clinically with Yale New Haven Hospital. She works as a nurse practitioner weekly at Trinity College Health Center. Grossman has presented and written multiple national and regional presentations and publications in the areas of her research on leadership, evidence-based practice, pathophysiology, geriatrics, primary and critical care patient outcome studies, and nursing education. She is a past member of the Connecticut State Board of Nursing and a member of Sigma Theta Tau International Mu Chi Chapter, American Critical Care Nurses Association, the National Organization of Nurse Practitioner Faculty, the Academy of Nurse Practitioners, and the American Nurses Association.

Mentoring in Nursing

A Dynamic and Collaborative Process

Sheila C. Grossman, PhD, APRN-BC

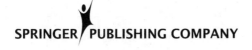

SPRINGER PUBLISHING COMPANY

New York

Springer Publishing Company, LLC.
11 West 42nd Street
New York, NY 10036
www.springerpub.com

Acquisitions Editor: Sally J. Barhydt
Production Editor: Gail F. Farrar
Cover design: Joanne E. Honigman
Composition: Publishers' Design and Production Services, Inc.

07 08 09 10 / 5 4 3 2 1

Library of Congress Cataloging-in-Publication Data

Grossman, Sheila.
   Mentoring in nursing : a dynamic and collaborative process / Sheila C. Grossman. — 1st ed.
      p. ; cm.
   Includes bibliographical references and index.
   ISBN-13: 978-0-8261-5385-2
   ISBN-10: 0-8261-5385-2
   1. Mentoring in nursing.   2. Nursing-Study and teaching (Preceptorship)   I. Title.
   [DNLM: 1. Mentors.   2. Nursing.   3. Interpersonal Relations. WY 18 G878m 2007]
RT86.45.G7647 2007
610.73—dc22

                                                                                        2006051251

Printed in the United States of America by Bang Printing.

Contents

Preface

The intent of this book is to help nurses, educators, administrators, and nursing students change the ways nurses do things, frequently separately from others and always in the same lock-step structured manner, to become empowered by developing a mentoring spirit in the nursing profession, and to facilitate a mentoring culture where encouragement, recognition, and respect are the predominant themes.

Nurses who feel that little is right at their work setting, who are interested in developing their leadership ability and empowering themselves, and who are interested in obtaining recognition for their work, their unit or department, agency, or institution should read this book. Anyone interested in joining the mentoring culture of nursing who feels she or he can be encouraging to others and has the potential to change the health care setting into a high-performance, yet caring, environment will benefit from this book.

Mentoring in Nursing: A Dynamic and Collaborative Process provides multiple ideas regarding the process of mentoring and how nurses can do great things for themselves and their profession. The literature base for the book includes a broad range of resources that discuss the process of mentoring and its outcomes. Mentoring can assist people in being better than what they would be solely by themselves. Once a mentee becomes self-empowered, there is a greater likelihood of being more creative, better able to adjust to changes, to be visionary, to manage conflict effectively, to take risks, to communicate effectively, and to be a critical thinker. It is evident that the closeness that develops between mentors and mentees sparks energy and creativity that assist individuals in maximizing their talents.

Chapter 1 defines the process of mentoring, the evolution of mentoring, types of mentoring, components and stages of the process, rationale for the contemporary process of mentoring, characteristics of classic mentoring, advantages and disadvantages of the process, additional support roles of the process, and research findings to support the need for mentoring. Chapter 2 relates how nurses have begun to develop a mentoring culture, best practices regarding mentoring in nursing, culturally competent mentoring, and examples of developing mentoring experiences in nursing. Chapter 3 discusses the concept of empowerment; strategies to help empower oneself, others, and the profession; a comparison of empowerment with the enabling process; and how creating a mentoring culture will further empower the profession. Chapter 4 analyzes characteristics of effective mentors, mentees, and mentoring. It stresses that one size, or type, of mentoring program does not necessarily fit all needs.

Chapter 5 describes methods for capturing the role of an effective mentor; delineates characteristics of effective mentors, preceptors, and coaches; and identifies benefits for those who participate in some form of mentoring. Chapter 6 discusses effective mentee relationships, ideas for choosing an effective mentor or mentors, suggestions for maximizing one's potential for being chosen by an effective mentor, and both the benefits and possible negatives of being in a mentoring relationship. Chapter 7 presents outcome implications related to mentoring for the profession, the organization, and patient consumers, mentors, and mentees. Chapter 8 summarizes the implications of what a mentoring culture will do for the profession of nursing, the organizations that employ nurses, and the mentors and mentees themselves.

Everyone has a part to play in a mentoring relationship, and it is a myth that only older and more experienced individuals can be mentors. Isn't it true that any form of energy can mentor or inspire us? So how many times have you encountered this energy? Have you perhaps missed some of these stimulating exchanges? Have you become so entrenched in your own agenda that you have lost contact with the network and have eventually become outside the network? So many talented people have been marginalized in their organizations due to the "outnetworked phenomenon." So how does one get back on track? *Mentoring in Nursing* was written to assist nurses in identifying how anyone who wants and is willing to can be renetworked into a successful mentoring relationship. Mentoring in nursing encompasses a guided experience, whether it be formally or informally assigned over a mutually agreed-on period of time that empowers the mentor and mentee to develop personally and professionally within a caring, collaborative, culturally competent, nonevaluated, and respectful environment.

The professional aspect is especially important because it needs to include not just what the mentoring can do for the mentee and the mentor but also what it can do for the nursing profession. Essentially the profession must foster a mentoring culture that offers networking to all who want to take advantage of it and are willing to give to it. Probably one of the best ways to get on track is to be part of a team that partners with other effective groups interested in similar outcomes, continually work on developing your leadership skills, and encourage others whom you interact with to do the same.

The major points in this book revolve around several themes:

- The importance of being more flexible in working with others and changing how we currently do some things
- The need to empower oneself to be a leader in order to make a difference
- Being able to create a mentoring spirit in nursing in which nurses will be recognized for their expertise

Mentoring is not a commodity that comes in a one-size-fits-all mentality; it must be individualized to each nurse according to his or her needs. The classic mentoring dyad has evolved to include multiple mentors and peer mentoring groups. Networking and partnering are imperative for organizational, professional, and individual success.

The profession stands to benefit greatly from the effects of a mentoring spirit in nursing. My hope is that nurses will be more satisfied with their work, fewer nurses will leave the profession, more nurses will enter, and fewer nurses will work in ways that can be destructive of young and new members of the profession. *Mentoring in Nursing: A Dynamic and Collaborative Process* is designed to help nurses in practice, administration, and educational roles understand the benefits of mentoring others as well as the value of being mentored themselves.

Acknowledgments

There are numerous students who participated as mentees in the Fairfield University School of Nursing Leadership Mentoring experiences as well as colleagues who served as mentors from all types of health care agencies in southwestern Connecticut who greatly facilitated the writing of this book. I extend my sincere appreciation to each of them and to all at the School of Nursing for their assistance with this project. Special thanks goes to Lydia Greiner, MS, APRN-BC, manager of community services, Fairfield University School of Nursing, for her assistance in helping both mentors and mentees. Great appreciation also goes to the Helene Fuld Foundation, which supported the mentoring project, and Fairfield University for granting me a sabbatical to write this book.

My gratitude is also extended to Grayce Sills, professor emeritus, Ohio State University, one of my first role models and a truly legendary mentor in nursing, for her wise and creative reflections in the Foreword of this book, and to Sally Barhydt, current editor, and Ruth Chasek, previous editor, at Springer Publishing Company, and Joyce Fitzpatrick, PhD, RN, FAAN for their assistance in publishing this book. I thank my many colleagues and friends who have mentored me over the years; my husband, Bob; and our daughters, Lisa and Beth, who have always supported me in everything I do. I also salute my sister, Ellen, who has consistently been the greatest mentor one could ever have.

Foreword

The twenty-first century is here. What is apparent is that much is required for all those who work in health care to do differently that which has always been done and to do it better. There are a host of reasons for this state of affairs. Two major paradigm shifts at work frame the challenges—challenges that make this book a guide as well as a compelling text for all those in the health care field who are struggling with the complexities of learning how to engage in the process of becoming a health care professional. I have deliberately broadened the discussion here to include more than nurses, inasmuch as the paradigm shifts are relevant to all who are learning how to become helping professionals in this rapidly changing world.

When I began in nursing more than 50 years ago, all I needed to know to become a successful nurse was taught and modeled by my elders. There was not even enough content to fill the 1065 days that constituted the time frame for diploma education of that era. We learned how to mix drugs and solutions and make suppositories since there was time left over when all there was to know in nursing had been taught. I relate this as an introduction to the two paradigm changes that frame those challenges.

The first paradigm was conceived by Margaret Mead, one of the intellectual giants of cultural anthropology. Mead developed the following explanatory paradigm for patterns of cultural learning. She postulated three patterns of cultural learning: postfigurative learning, cofigurative learning, and prefigurative learning. In postfigurative learning, children learn from adults, and all that is required for successful adulthood is to pattern after successful adults. That was my experience in the diploma program. In that era, there was very little change in the world of nursing and health care. I taught students as I had been taught. I modeled my practice after my head nurse who was a very good head nurse. I watched her and sometimes would ask questions, but for the most part I simply tried to emulate her behavior.

In some way, I absorbed values and beliefs that continue to inform my practice today. This is an example of postfigurative learning.

In the cofigurative pattern of learning, peers learn from peers—children learn from other children, for example. This occurs when the pace of change accelerates, and there is more to be known than was known in the world of the elders. For us in nursing, this period of accelerated knowledge development and technological advances required much change. Bright young nurses, especially in the area of critical care, began to teach their peers. Few of their elders had the requisite cutting-edge knowledge and skill to be successful in the environment of rapid change.

In the prefigurative pattern of learning, adults learn from children. When the pace of change rapidly accelerates, it is the young who first apprehend the present and the future. They must teach the elders what is needed in the present. This has been most apparent in the era of expanded electronic technology, which often defeats elders, who need the young to help them learn in this new world. This is the prefigurative pattern of learning.

It is important to remember that all three patterns of cultural learning are present all the time. It is the rate of change in the culture that determines the relative prevalence of each pattern. This book provides guidelines for mentoring relationships that reflect all three patterns of cultural learning. Indeed, all are needed in this era of enormous change and increased complexity.

In this new century, we are witnessing change at unprecedented speed. It is incumbent on all of us in the helping professions to be cognizant of the need for continued support and guidance by elders, but the elders must also listen and learn from the young, and the young must help each other if the profession's covenant with the public is to be kept.

The second paradigm change has occurred over the past 50 years and represents a mind shift from viewing the patient as someone to be done to and for, to a view of the patient as someone to be worked with, as in collaboration. The changed view of nursing is still well illustrated in the work of Nightingale and Virginia Henderson. However, as the world became more complex and there was more knowledge to bring to bear, a new model was needed. A new model emerged and was fueled by the seminal work of Hildegard Peplau. Nursing now was to be learned as an interpersonal process.

At about the same time, there began to be the first glimmer of the consumer movement in health care. The consumer movement, for us in nursing, was experienced as a challenge to visiting hours, as well as pressure for fathers to be present in delivery rooms, among many other changes.

The interpersonal paradigm shift also meant that nurses now had to focus on self-knowledge as well as how to work *with* patients and families.

This new skill to be learned was *collaboration*. Working with this concept has been and continues to be a major challenge for us in nursing. Many of us were taught to work for the cooperation of the patient. Cooperation meant that the patient willingly allowed us to do to and for him or her. Moreover, we hoped that the patient would be happy about this situation. The more difficult task is to engage the patient in a collaborative process. It is in the service of this needed learning that mentoring finds its central purpose.

At the heart of this book is the idea that the interpersonal relationship between mentor and mentee is essential to the process of learning. The book has many illustrations of all three types of cultural learning, all of them needed in this rapidly swirling whitewater culture of health care. This book is as much for the elders as it is for the young. The young need the re-membered history, the embedded values, and the rich store of wisdom of the elders. The wise ones need the voices of the young to tell them of the present so that they might discern together a future that neither alone can comprehend. The young need each other as well to share the joy of collab-orative work. When we learn this skill with each other, we can begin to find the echoes of that learning in collaborative work with colleagues, patients, and families. In this way, the challenge of the two major paradigm shifts can be answered.

It is my hope that anyone in any of the health care professions can find a road map in this book, a guide in an uncertain future—a future often only dimly apprehended that is waiting on the horizon. This future is waiting for the wisdom, the talents, the knowledge, and the caring of each generation to fulfill its promise.

For all who read this book, I wish you much joy as you go about ful-filling the promise of your generation.

Grayce M. Sills, PhD, RN, FAAN
Professor Emeritus
The Ohio State University
Director, OSU Harding
Collaborative for
Behavioral Health
Columbus, Ohio

CHAPTER 1

Mentoring

From a Classic Dyad to a Dynamic Network

M*entoring* is an elusive term that has existed for years in many disciplines and continues to evolve (Ehrich, Tennent, & Hansford, 2002). Although there have been various definitions of the term, the general purpose of mentoring has been similar in its many usages and is frequently described as dynamic and applicable to the professional and personal development of a less experienced, young individual—the mentee (Roberts, 2000). Certainly mentoring is not a new phenomenon, and it will undoubtedly continue to evolve from a hierarchical to a more collaborative process. McWeeny (2002), recognizing that there is an expanding conception of the mentoring process, likens it to a changing mosaic and says, "We are moving from a dyad model to more inclusive, diverse and enduring models" (p. 4). In today's world, it seems only sensible that mentoring will evolve from a one-on-one relationship to a network with the overwhelming focus on team effort. With the expansion of telecommunication technology, the mentoring process has expanded to include a global networking infrastructure of mentor-mentee linking.

This chapter describes the process of mentoring; the evolution of mentoring; types, components, and stages of the process; a rationale for the contemporary process of mentoring; characteristics of classic mentoring; advantages and disadvantages of the process; additional support roles of the process, and research findings to support the need for mentoring. Certainly the lack of consensus over the definition of *mentoring* presents definitional issues for researchers in all disciplines. I hope that descriptions of mentoring from disciplines outside nursing will increase understanding regarding how mentoring has developed in the nursing profession to support the following definition:

> Mentoring in nursing encompasses a guided, nonevaluated experience, formal or informal, assigned over a mutually agreed-on period of time that empowers the mentor and mentee to develop personally and professionally within the auspices of a caring, collaborative, and respectful environment.

THE PROCESS OF MENTORING

Most of the research that has been published on mentoring is in business and education; therefore, this chapter presents concepts that have come from studies in disciplines that have influenced how nursing has used mentoring (Bell, 1998; Daloz, 1999; Gay, 1994; Johnson & Huwe, 2003; Kram, 1983, 1986; Levinson, Darrow, Klein, Levinson, & McKee, 1978; Luna & Cullen, 1996; Murray, 2001; Roberts, 2000; Schweibert, 2000; Shea, 1997; Carew, 1998; Sinetar, 1998). The term *mentoring* is thought to be an offspring of human living, teaching and learning, giving and receiving wisdom in all relationships, leadership, and succession (Huang & Lynch, 1995).

Some feel a mentorship involves just two people, while others feel a mentorship can be a group of people helping each other. This perspective reinforces the more contemporary idea that it is generally more worthwhile to reach out to, network with, encourage, and mentor others than to work solo. However, although many people recommend a mentorship, there are successful individuals who routinely work on their own. They manage each heartache and organizational burden alone just as they also receive merit and fame for their accomplishments alone. Even leaders generally want mentors (or at least friends with the mentor's spirit) because they are "reaching into the unknown for self expression" and could use some encouragement (Sinetar, 1998, p. 39). Can't everyone use some encouragement? Isn't success sweeter when it is a result of a team effort? Why not extend the classic dyadic mentoring definition to include collaborating within a larger group of people with the purpose of creating a mentoring spirit in work groups?

Today's work setting demands its workers to produce outcomes that are measurable, cost-effective, and make a difference. It stands to reason that these demands would be more easily reached if workers teamed up with others and shared their various strengths to generate more productivity. However, it may not be as easy as it sounds. One has to imagine or, in some cases, remember, how challenging it is to motivate others, which is extremely difficult, and sometimes impossible to do. The other part of this idea of a collaborative mentoring network has to include the fact that most people do not give unless they are going to be receiving or getting something back for themselves. So perhaps it is important to reflect on how mentoring evolved and came to be what it is today: a process of facilitating one's colleague's as well as one's own success.

Historically, most have thought the term was derived from *The Odyssey* where the Greek poet, Homer, wrote about the wise mentor who was assigned to protect the king's son in his absence. Andrews and Wallis (1999) correct this erroneously defined identification to say the origin of the modern mentor is actually from *Les Aventures de Telemaque*, by Fenelon (1699/1994). This perception seems to be far from what mentoring has evolved to today, but in a way, it is not so different because one of the roles of a mentor is to do just that: protect the mentee from nurses who destroy other nurses, the "sharks" in the profession or organization. Who hasn't known a shark in the nursing profession? How many times have nurses been accused of not assisting the new and young nurses entering the profession? Contemporary literature such as *The Lion King* with Zazu and *Star Wars* with Yoda also reflect mentor characters and portray stories we can all relate to in our past.

People enjoy hearing about how someone has succeeded and tend to be proud of how their influence, no matter how small, may have helped in this effort. Zey (1990) interviewed 150 executives from Fortune 500 corporations and found mentoring to be the most important reason that an individual was successful—even more so than academic credentials. The truth of this fact is reinforced in our profession, in which many of today's successful nurses have their educational roots from a diploma to a doctoral program, but have climbed the corporate ladder in either service or higher education as they made more connections. It seems that these connections among nurses and with other health care providers begun in early stages of one's profession are what makes certain individuals more successful in their careers.

Murray (2001) has developed and refined, over a 30-year period, the Facilitated Mentoring Model and defines *mentoring* as a process of assigning a more skilled with a less skilled person with the goal of increasing the skills of the mentee. However, over 30 years, the model has evolved to reflect that learning, growth, and skill development occur with the mentor as well. Murray introduces concepts such as total quality, self-managed work teams, and facilitated mentoring and asks people in business to be more open to networking with others, with the idea that a team is more successful than an individual. Using these quality improvement methods can foster new ways of mentoring, such as networking with high performers as outside consultants, finding out new ideas from interacting with peers from one's professional organizations, and hiring a specific consulting group or individual to come in and teach an identified needed skill. Joiner (1994) emphasizes the importance of promoting collaborative interaction but also notes that each individual must be fully accountable for a part of the work. He states that having a productive group versus just one individual working solo is key to "delighting the customer and not just satisfying them." This rationale can be applied to health care delivery success, where patient satisfaction outcomes are continually being monitored and where a broader view of staff mentoring could be helpful.

Many of those in the workforce today, especially those between 30 and 40 years old, are not seeking a one-employer long-term career; rather, they seek out multiple employment opportunities. They believe that in order to accelerate their career, they need to have multiple employers. Most employees today do not have the blind loyalty of their predecessors and want to be recognized for their individual expertise. They expect to advance their careers by working in a variety of work settings, which can facilitate a much broader network of mentors that can propel their careers.

Schwiebert (2000) describes mentoring as "a phenomenon of modern times" (p. ix), a life-changing dynamic and ever-evolving process. Mentoring constitutes more than being a product of the "good ole boy circle." Simon and Eby (2003) define mentoring as a relationship that allows junior members of a group an opportunity to receive guidance, advice, and "opportunities for personal and professional development" (p. 1083). The mentor too will reap career rewards from participating in the mentoring. The potential opportunities gained from networking through a successful mentorship appear to be key for professional career growth. Although this "good ole boy" concept is present in the nursing profession, it is not accurate to think it is the only reason someone succeeds. It seems that having the right mentor who might be in the right circle of successful leaders who mentors extremely well is most beneficial for mentee success.

So what is success? In nursing, it can include a variety of achievements such as

- certification in one's area of specialty;
- becoming an Advanced Practice Registered Nurse;
- promotion to the highest clinical ladder;
- obtaining grant funding;
- achieving a top administrative position in practice or academia;

- election to lead a national or international professional organization;
- appointment to a prestigious board;
- selection as a Fellow of the American Academy of Nursing (FAAN).

Achieving one of these milestones is a life-changing dynamic and, in the majority of instances is due to an ever-evolving process of networking with colleagues and receiving mentoring from advisers, role models, teachers, and others. Nurses interested in gaining these honors need to connect with others, and this needs to occur several times each year.

Shea (1999) says mentoring is a "developmental caring, sharing and helping relationship where one person invests time, know-how, and effort in enhancing another person's growth, knowledge and skills" (p. 3). This may be a good universal definition because no mention is made of who matched the two people, no time limit is stated, and it allows both mentor and mentee to assist each other without the evaluation component hindering self-expression and growth for the sake of personal growth. However, it needs to be expanded to include more of a network of experts. Furthermore, Shea defines a mentor as "anyone who has an important, long-lasting beneficial life or style enhancing effect on another person, generally as a result of personal one-on-one contact—and this relationship goes beyond one's duty or fulfilling one's obligations" (p. 3). A mentee is "a person being mentored by another person or persons; especially one who makes an effort to assess, internalize and use effectively the knowledge, skills, insights, perspectives, or wisdom offered by the mentor(s)" (p. 3). He further suggests there is a spectrum of mentor-mentee interactions (see Figure 1.1) that can be displayed on a horizontal continuum, with a formal program (a structured program that meets the organization's goals) on the extreme left of the continuum, an informal relationship (interpersonal connection between mentor and mentee for the mentor to help the mentee in specific areas) in the middle, and on the extreme right side of the continuum situational responses. Situational responses are isolated incidents of specific advising by an experienced or knowledgeable individual to meet another individual's needs. The formal aspect of this framework includes evaluation of the mentee, so this aspect of the model seems to be more akin to that of a preceptor, not a mentor.

| Formal Program | $\longrightarrow$ | Informal Relationship | $\longrightarrow$ | Situational Responses |

FIGURE 1.1   **Spectrum of mentor/mentee interactions.**

EVOLUTION OF THE MENTORING PROCESS

Wickman and Sjodin (1997), Shea (1997), and Bell (1998) describe mentoring as an evolving mosaic. Examples of mentoring in situational, informal, formal, individual, group, and forum scenarios are discussed. The ultimate purpose of each of their books is to show that mentoring increases productivity and accelerates individual and organizational goal accomplishment. All ascribe to the traditional definition of mentoring as a process by which an experienced person assists a less experienced one to attain his or her goals. However, they too expand and reframe the classic mentoring process by describing other activities that assist less experienced individuals as well as mentors to achieve their goals. Group mentoring versus the traditional one-on-one relationship is compared and contrasted to show that group mentoring decreases the likelihood of mismatches between the mentor and mentee, utilizes the mentor's time and expertise more wisely, allows for a greater impact on more employees, supports collaborative team building, builds peer networks, and allows for vertical mentor-mentee and mentee-mentor mentoring.

COMPONENTS OF THE MENTORING PROCESS

The less skilled person in the classic mentoring relationship is called a *mentee, protégé,* or *novice,* whereas the more experienced is always called a *mentor.* In order for the mentoring to be successful, Lee (2000) suggests that the mentor have a strong belief that the mentee has the capacity to succeed. Motivation and empowerment generate mentoring where both the mentor and mentee share their skills. In order to have an effective mentoring relationship, the mentor must try to remove obstacles, give emotional support, and allow for recognition of achievement in the work setting. In this way, mentees are supported to work harder to achieve their goals and ultimately achieve higher self-esteem as well. Being motivated to do a good job empowers the nurse, and this power makes her feel motivated and gives her the confidence to accomplish her goals and gain increased self-esteem. The classic mentoring process is generally thought of as a relationship of two people: one (the mentee) who is a young and inexperienced person with great promise and the other who is a successful leader (the mentor) in the mentee's professional area. The mentor advises, teaches, coaches, role-models, and connects the mentee to significant networks. Additionally, the mentee often needs to be able to offer a new skill set, resources, or some connection to the relationship that will benefit the mentor. Kram (1986), a foremost mentoring expert, identifies three primary components that are most frequently part of a mentorship in Table 1.1.

The psychosocial aspect includes assisting a person to acclimate to an organization's culture, suggesting hints for balancing work and personal life, whereas career focuses involve networking, providing strategies for accomplishing goals for career advancement, and new professional endeavors. Some mentoring relationships consist of assisting the mentee with personal development issues such as balancing family and career, moving to the right neighborhood, socializing with the politically correct crowd, dressing for the part, and vacationing at the correct places. These mentoring dyads tended to be long-term relationships that last for an extended period of time, or even forever. The mentor and mentee become friends and share a great amount of time together. Other mentorships leave the personal development area to the mentee to gain from others. The idea of developing trust between the mentor and mentee that increases with time is a significant part of the relationship, since it allows for support and sharing of experiences. The mentor's job includes career functions, such as sponsorship, coaching, protection, and exposure, while the psychosocial role involves role modeling, counseling, acceptance, confirmation, and friendship. Kram (1983) points out that not all of these functions may be appropriate in some organizations or with some individuals, but clarifies that a mentorship should include focusing on psychosocial as well as advising on steps for career advancement. It is not uncommon for a mentor and mentee to identify specific outcomes they expect to gain from the relationship. In some settings, contracts are developed that set out the expectations of each party.

TABLE 1.1   **Primary Components of a Mentorship**

1. Career defined, which focuses on advancement in the organization by a mentor's coaching, connecting the mentee to networks, protecting the mentee, and giving challenging assignments to the mentee

2. Psychosocial functions, which increase the mentee's self-worth, competence, identity, and general effectiveness by receiving friendship and counseling from the mentor

3. Role modeling by the mentor so there is someone for the mentee to identify with and emulate

RATIONALES FOR THE EMERGENCE
OF CONTEMPORARY MENTORING

Human resource departments have been singing the praises of mentoring since the 1950s. When management clarified how important it was for employees to be tied to the organization and be loyal for the good of the organization, more and more employees were tagged as fitting into the culture or not. Administration was interested in cloning the "good ones," and this is where specific plans were instituted in business corporations that assigned new employees to the good, experienced employees who fit into the culture. Malcolm Knowles (1984), a master adult educator, wrote about how adults learn and can relearn at any age. Business models coach new employees to become effective executives. Mentees can gain increased knowledge from their assigned mentors. Educators began to change their philosophy of spoon-feeding their students to a more self-directed emphasis whereby the learner assumed more responsibility for learning (Cross, 1981). This included the idea of setting up shadowing experiences with experts and having internships in which learners could practice their skills. Lifelong learning triggered a self-development type of philosophy in which individuals were guided to become more performance centered versus content focused. This paradigm change influenced educators to set up learning experiences in which the student had exposure to and practice time in the work he or she wanted to do after graduation. Given that the educator could not be in two places at the same time, students were assigned to work with individuals who worked in the specific area in which students needed experience. As such, the precepting model used in nursing, pharmacy, medicine, and other professional training programs was instituted.

Restifo and Yoder (2004) describe classic mentoring as a long-term involvement between two individuals paired up by a supervisor. The mentor tends to be the person with advanced job-related experience, knowledge, and power in their organization. The mentor is believed to facilitate the mentee in developing skills and acquiring networks and organizational savvy that is so crucial for survival as well as success in any profession. Others argue (Weil, 2001; Sinetar, 1998) that these relationships evolve over time, are spontaneous and not assigned, and tend to be critical for leadership succession in any profession. So it seems there is disagreement as to whether mentoring must evolve over time or exist for a specified time period, whether a mentoring dyad is supposed to be assigned or can constitute a spontaneous connection, and whether mentors should formally evaluate a mentee. The emergence of new mentoring models, such as multiple mentors, the junior partner mentoring the senior individual, and peer mentoring networks, are all products of the classic mentor-mentee dyad.

TYPES OF MENTORING

Multiple Mentoring

Mentoring is a complex relationship between two people, and the process is even more complex when the mentee, mentor, or both are involved in more than one mentoring relationship. This simultaneous mentoring involvement, called *multiple mentoring*, has become more common as the Internet and communication technology have allowed more global and quick connections. For example, in a multiple mentoring model, the mentee can seek out advice from more than one mentor as well as use the most qualified mentor for each need. *Reverse mentoring* is when a senior person receives mentoring from a junior person or the mentor is mentored by the mentee. An example of this reverse mentoring follows:

> Susan, a doctoral student, has begun a mentorship with Dr. Theng, who studies the concept of hardiness in chronic illness. Susan has been receiving hints and suggestions, such as: which conferences to submit abstracts for presentation, whether to submit for a paper or poster presentation, ideas on power point and poster development, and strategies for being chosen to keynote a conference or be a part of a symposium or panel, and has even been connected to Dr. Theng's collegial network as she prepares for a presentation she is doing with Dr. Theng at a national conference. Susan suggests to Dr. Theng that they incorporate Web enhancement technology in the presentation. Dr. Theng is not familiar with Starboard Technology, and so Susan shares her expertise with her mentor. Dr. Theng is elated with the results and has Susan assist her in making these applications to all of her class presentations. Susan also has 10 years working as a diabetic teaching nurse and five years of experience working as a family nurse practitioner. She has access to all patient data files in the clinic, which includes over 6000 chronically ill people. She is still a per diem practitioner at this clinic and has received Institutional Review Board consent to study hardiness with diabetics. Using this database, she is going to be working as the primary researcher with Dr. Theng as a co-investigator.

This example portrays the give-and-take relationship that often occurs in nursing in which most individuals have clinical expertise and a network in an area prior to returning for a higher degree. They come to the mentoring relationship to gain knowledge and experience in administration, education, or research.

Peer and Co-Mentoring

Co-mentoring or peer mentoring is dependent on mutual trust similar to traditional mentoring; however, it differs greatly with regard to equality. Since there is no hierarchical relationship, the colleagues must be extremely trustworthy of each other so that neither of them derives more or less from the connection. Rymer (2002) and Sinetar (1998) reinforce the significance of each individual having equal roles in peer mentoring. It is a myth that only elders or organizational superiors can be mentors. In fact, Sinetar (1998) goes as far as to say that any virtuous energy, from a friend, a child, or an idea, can mentor or inspire us. All of these models assist with acclimating mentees to their job and advancing their career path, as well as helping their mentor's career. With the multiple mentoring and reverse mentoring models, there can be horizontal and vertical mentoring going on simultaneously, depending on a variety of beneficial and mitigating factors.

An example of this includes Sue's (1981) Minority Identity Model, which explains how minorities progress through five psychosocial stages of cultural identity development as they work with a mentor:

1. Conformity. The individual tends to be self-deprecating and relates to his or her own culture.
2. Dissonance. The person is developing some conflict with the culture.
3. Resistance and immersion. The individual is more self-deprecating and is rejecting the dominant society.
4. Introspection. There is much self-evaluation and reflection for the dominant society and how the person is interacting.
5. Synergism and awareness. The individual can accept his or her own cultural identity but also develops a selective appreciation of the culture in which he or she is currently immersed.

So what are the implications of these stages to mentoring? It depends where the individual is in identity development; thus, mentees have different needs depending on what stage they are experiencing. This can be compounded if the mentor and the mentee are of the same culture but are in different stages of the identity model. This is where the mentor will need to role-model well regarding the importance for a mentee to find or develop his or her own style and not conform to the style of another. It is important to be aware of the issue of cultural diversity and to try to use the developmental framework already noted or a similar model to educate both the mentor and mentee so appropriate networking and advisement can be ensured. If a structured mentoring program is in effect, it is helpful to have opportunities for culturally diverse individuals to be involved so that there can be maximized networking with others.

Schwiebert (2000) indicates there are not enough mentors for all who seek one, especially for culturally diverse individuals. She points out that there are many mentors who practice alterity, which is the perpetuation of a monocultural concept of mentoring. It is when one person truly believes that anyone outside his or her own culture is strange or inferior, and so feels that he or she should set the standards for all people. This would obviously thwart mentoring success for many individuals, especially those from minority groups. It is not known if pairing mentor and mentee with a similar cultural background has the optimum outcome. Depending on the awareness of the mentor, there could be serious misunderstandings transferred to the mentee, which can often result from insensitivity and ignorance (Schwiebert, 2000). The question remains, If no culturally similar mentor can be found for a mentee, is it better to have no mentor or one from a different culture? Further research on transcultural mentoring is necessary in all disciplines.

CHARACTERISTICS OF THE CLASSIC MENTORING RELATIONSHIP

Wilson and Elman (1990) believe that mentoring is the most successful way to pass along the "norms, values, assumptions, and myths that are central to an organization's survival" (p. 93). As a dynamic process, mentoring is continuing to evolve, so it becomes easier for important legacies and an organization's values to be passed on to the next generation. So too with a nursing mentor-mentee relationship, the values or beliefs of the profession can be preserved.

The classic, formal mentoring dyad generally lasts for about 5–10 years (Kram, 1986; Levinson et al., 1978). Informal mentoring is spontaneous and nonassigned, whereas long-term mentoring is assigned and generally lasts for a short period of time until the mentee or preceptee learns the skills to assume a job. Kram (1986) found that with formal mentoring, there is more superficiality between mentor and mentee than in an informal relationship.

Wickman and Sjodin (1996) describe many interesting accounts of their mentoring relationship, which lasted about 5 years in which Wickman was generally the mentor and Sjodin was generally the mentee. Their book, *Mentoring: The Most Obvious Yet Overlooked Key to Achieving More in Life Than You Ever Dreamed Possible*, is helpful in explaining exactly how to go about getting a mentor or advising someone else interested in obtaining a mentor as well as strategies for maximizing the benefits of a mentoring relationship.

STAGES OF THE MENTORING PROCESS

Kram (1983) studied mentor-mentee pairs in a longitudinal study in business and found similarities between the pairs that helped her identify phases of the mentoring process. She found most relationships averaged 5 years in length and consisted of four stages. Others have validated this research in both business (Pollock, 1995) and education settings (Johnson & Huwe, 2003). There are five most commonly viewed stages of the mentoring process:

1. Initiation stage. The senior person is admired, and the junior person is considered coachable, and a general getting-to-know-each-other time begins.
2. Cultivation stage. The mentee is at the peak of development, sets goals, and gains self-esteem, and generally works on both professional and personal goal achievement.
3. Separation stage. The junior person starts to express independence. It is a time of anxiety when the junior person separates from the senior person. The intensity in the relationship begins to decrease considerably.
4. Redefinition stage. There is a collegial relationship that allows for more equality between the mentee and the mentor. The mentee may feel abandoned, depending on where he or she is developmentally. It is the time that most feel the relationship is no longer needed or desired, or it becomes a more peer-like relationship (Kram, 1983).

These stages of mentoring portray a cyclic process or a continuum that is based on the individual's developmental stages as he or she matures in the relationship. Depending on where one is in one's life and career, one will generally be either mentoring someone, be mentored, or be in a network that co-mentors one another. When one reviews stages of the mentoring process, it is most common to think of Kram's (1983) universal stages.

However, it might be important to also factor into this framework the idea that mentors may mentor differently depending on where they are in the development of their mentoring skills. Most mentors are made, not born, and that is why it is interesting to review Bennis's framework. Mentoring is part of being a leader, and similar to developing one's leadership ability, one will need to build mentoring skills.

Bennis (2004) likens the stages that leaders go through to the seven ages of man as described by Shakespeare in *As You Like It*. Bennis describes the mentoring a leader experiences as the leader evolves:

Stage 1, Infant Executive.   It is crucial that during this stage, the infant executive has a mentor. Bennis says that a mentor has attributes of both male and female gender, which points to the potential richness of the relationship and suggests that a mentor relationship is deeper than just a teacher and student. In reality "mentors do not materialize on their own" (p. 48); rather, the best mentors are "usually recruited." A characteristic of a true leader is having the ability to "identify, woo, and win the mentors who will change his/her life" (p. 48). This is comparable to the ability of being as skillful as an experienced head-hunter who gets a client placed.

Stage 2, Schoolboy With Shining Face.   The new leader should "make a low-key entry" while he or she learns the culture and benefits from the wisdom of those already there. It is imperative for a mentee to "establish [being] open to contributions of others."

Stage 3, Lover, With a Woeful Ballad.   This is the time when one needs to separate from colleagues as friends since they are no longer one's peers. It becomes crucial to delegate.

Stage 4, Beautiful Soldier.   The mentor may become too comfortable with role. The mentor should be sure to nurture his or her shining stars, but not take from them without due recognition.

Stage 5, General, Full of Wise Saws.   It is crucial to hear both the good and the bad and to act accordingly.

Stage 6, Statesman With Spectacles on Nose.   It is here one should do more mentoring since this is when a leader's power base wanes.

Stage 7, Sage, Second Childishness.   This is where having mentored throughout one's career will pay off. It is the professional equivalent of having grandchildren and leaving a legacy for future generations.

Bennis says each stage of leadership a person experiences in life brings new crises and challenges, and that having experienced these stages, one then knows what to expect and this knowledge helps one help not only oneself but also others to get through life's challenges. Similarly, one can envision how a nurse would follow various mentors' steps during his or her nursing career.

ADVANTAGES AND DISADVANTAGES OF MENTORING

Many (Bell, 1998; Bennetts, 2000; Sinetar, 1998) identify benefits for the mentee, mentor, and organization, including

- quicker learning curves for mentee and mentor;
- increased communication of corporate values;
- reduced turnover at a time when new recruits may be difficult to locate;
- increased loyalty;
- improved one-on-one communication and team spirit within work groups;
- increased employee productivity;
- added time for oneself to work on one's own goals;
- added information from mentees regarding what is going on outside your department;
- creation of allies in the mentees for the future.

These advantages are helpful to the mentor, mentee, organization, and the profession. Peluchette and Jeanquart (2000) describe the impact mentors have by connecting students and novices to the correct person for career success. Another advantage for mentors is that by mentoring, they develop increased credibility in the organization (Gilley & Boughton, 1996). One can gain credibility by delegating work appropriately, providing specific and timely performance feedback, helping employees identify work objectives for improvement, and demonstrating acceptable professional behavior.

Sinetar (1998) warns there are disadvantages of mentoring if "unhealthy mentors" attempt to manipulate mentees. Certainly it is possible for mentors to treat mentees without dignity and respect. Although the mentors may appear ultra-aggressive and confident, usually these mentors are intimidated and have very low self-esteem. Therefore, these types of individuals should be quickly identified as not to be used as mentors who are actually in need of a mentor—or at least guidance—for themselves. People who are this insecure at a later stage of their career may not be candidates for participating in a mentoring partnership since they cannot share and will do too much harm to their mentor or their mentee and themselves. There are also individuals who have been mentored and helped along the way who do not have any realization of it at all, or at least cannot admit that they have been mentored and have not climbed the ladder solely on their own. These individuals should not be tapped as mentors either.

There are other disadvantages as well, such as personality incompatibility, power-mongering mentors, and situations in which mentors are resentful of the mentee and make trouble for the mentee that can sabotage his or her career. Simon and Eby (2003) present findings that provide a description of negative mentoring experiences that they have collected. These relationships can vary in severity and frequency and may be characterized by minor obstructionism (e.g., not returning phone calls), hostility (e.g., talking negatively about someone behind his or her back), or serious overt aggression (e.g., physical attack). Possessiveness, jealousy, credit taking, deceit, and abuse, both psychological and physical, can occur in mentoring relationships.

ADDITIONAL SUPPORT ROLES INVOLVED IN MENTORING

There are multiple perceptions of what the role of a mentor and mentee involves and what the differences are between a preceptor/preceptee or coach/apprentice relationship and the mentor/mentee roles. Mentoring is very different from coaching (training for a project or being on a task force), role modeling (this occurs often without any relationship between two individuals and often the role model does not know someone thinks he or she is a role model), or consulting (generally an outsider who is paid to do a part of a project or coordinate a project).

The roles are used interchangeably. Certainly everyone knows that the essence of what is being referred to here is that one person advises and coaches another person. "Mentoring or coaching allows tired, disenchanted, and bored managers the opportunity to guide employees through the perils of organizational life like a lighthouse that shines the way for ships at night, steering them away from danger" (Gilley & Boughton, 1996, p. 171). So why is it necessary to operationally define mentoring, precepting, coaching, shadowing, or role modeling? Perhaps by defining these roles, people can have a better understanding as to what type of guided experience would best fit the circumstances of the situation. Also, it seems prudent to provide a discussion of what is actually known about all of these terms, and perhaps then research can further validate each concept so more appropriate guided experiences can be arranged for those who may or may not be able to experience a classic mentoring relationship.

Precepting

Preceptorships are an assigned relationship in which an experienced nurse assists in orienting a new employee, who is often referred to as an apprentice or, in some organizations, a preceptee (Flynn, 1997). Precepting is also the format used when a student is assigned to a teacher, nurse, or some other experienced professional to teach this person as well as evaluate aspects of his or her role. In nursing, a senior student generally has a preceptor in the clinical area that he or she is assigned to work with for approximately 160 hours in the student's final semester. The student follows the preceptor's schedule and works in a one-to-one relationship for a specific amount of time. The student has a faculty member who makes regular visits to assess how the preceptee is doing and discusses the student's performance with the preceptor on a routine basis. The preceptor is responsible to evaluate the student on a pass/fail checklist and reviews this with the student and faculty at the end of the required number of hours in the preceptorship. Experiential learning has been the mainstay of professional internships in most disciplines and used as a major pedagogy to teach not only the professional practice skills but also how to communicate and affect change in one's practice (Kolb, 1984).

Coaching

One function of a mentor is to coach the mentee by keeping the mentee aware of the politics in the organization, being supportive of the person's ideas, and acting as a sounding board when the mentee needs to discuss how to overcome weaknesses. Gilley and Boughton (1996) say the key to maximizing organizational performance is to have work environments that allow for increased self-esteem of all employees and provide not only organizational goal accomplishment but also personal growth and development. Coaching can be defined as comprising four roles: training, career coaching, confronting, and mentoring. The most important of these to the organization is the confronter role, which includes learning to be assertive, managing conflict, and collaborating to solve organizational problems. The faculty person is the coach in the student-preceptor-coach triangle and is responsible for obtaining the correct experiences and opportunities so that the student can accomplish individual and program goals.

Boreen and Niday (2003) also suggest the notion of self-mentoring or coaching oneself toward growth that others may refer to as auto-mentoring. Strategies used are reflection techniques, motivational self-talk, questioning, listening, critical thinking, and risk taking. Keeping weekly logs of positive and negative occurrences, discussing different ways to handle negative incidents, and implementing these new strategies assist the self-mentoring process. It is also important to have a network of peers to bounce ideas and share solutions for negative experiences. Self-reflection assists individuals to increase self-awareness and reprioritize their needs in order to maximize growth. Boreen and Niday report findings from the most recent (2003) National Commission on Teaching in America's Future Report that there are not enough good teachers. Mentoring has proven to be one of the most effective ways to keep teachers in the field, and this is thought to be true in the nursing profession as well.

Role Modeling

In shadowing or role modeling, there is generally an aspect of closeness between the role model and individual, although it is not uncommon for the role model to be totally unaware that someone is actually seeing him or her as a role model. Each of these role-modeling relationships has a place in assisting individuals to grow both professionally and personally. Role modeling is defined as extremely important in order to succeed with human adaptation (Kolb, 1984). It assists learning by offering behaviors that the less experienced person can imitate. Many times this imitation is specific to one type of behavior that a role model exemplifies. Other times people imitate role models for a general look or response that they perceive would be helpful to adapt in their own professional and personal growth. Experiential learning has been the mainstay of professional internships in most disciplines and used as a major pedagogy to teach not only the professional practice skills but also how to communicate and effect change in one's practice (Kolb, 1984).

Co-Mentoring

Peers, peer pals, co-mentors, and *buddies* are terms given for collaborative mentoring relationships between peers. These groups of colleagues are generally noncompetitive and are willing to network with each other to accomplish mutually agreed-on goals.

Daloz (1999) describes an individual's education as a transformational journey affected by mentor guides who model, offer a map, conceptualize, and provide a mirror. He correlates mentoring with teaching in that few teachers ever have the privilege of following a student through the entire journey but instead tend to accompany students along some parts of their journey.

Miller (2002) describes various examples of co-mentoring, interning, role modeling, and coaching. He presents two case studies depicting mentoring with Deloitte & Touche and Merrill Lynch's Scholarship Builder Program. He believes that mentoring in the business world is seen as important as work experience in an employee's career development and that it will continue to be appreciated even if a mentor and mentee are not in close geographic proximity. Telementoring and e-mail mentoring are becoming common tools used especially among peer networks and multiple mentoring relationship in business.

RESEARCH TO SUPPORT OUTCOMES OF MENTORING

Levinson et al. (1978) were the first educators to study outcomes of mentoring. Their findings include the importance of the mentor's believing in the mentee, sharing parts of the mentee's dream, and giving the dream his or her blessing. By doing this, they feel it helped to "define the mentee's newly emerging self" (p. 98).

The psychosocial theory of development (Erikson, 1963) suggests that the final stage of generativity correlates with the concept of mentoring because it allows all who have a concern for improving the world to participate by mentoring younger generations. Luna and Cullen (1996) suggest that this framework fits well in academia, where senior faculty mentor junior faculty to develop younger colleagues' talent and, at the same time, promote the department and university as well. Essentially generativity is "the building block of mentoring as one gives back or mentors a new generation" (Luna & Cullen, p. 18).

Roberts (2000) conducted a literature review of mentoring using a phenomenological approach. He defines mentoring as "a formalized process whereby a more knowledgeable and experienced person takes on a supportive role of overseeing and encouraging reflection and learning with a less experienced and knowledgeable person, so as to facilitate that person's career and personal development" (p. 162). Results of his literature review on mentoring research published between 1978 and 1999 demonstrated a consensus regarding the following themes as being components of the mentoring process:

- Supportive relationship
- Helping process
- Teaching learning process

- Reflective process
- Career development process
- Formalized process
- Mentoring process consisting of coaching, sponsoring, role modeling, and assessing
- Informal pairing of mentor and mentee

Research validates that people who have worked successfully with a mentor have more promotions, increased incomes, increased career satisfaction, and increased mobility than those without mentors (Schwiebert, 2000). The key to successful mentoring is collegiality and caring between the mentor, the mentee, and others in the organization. (Jarvis, 1992; Kram, 1983). Kram believes that mentees (in academia and business) can advance even more if multiple mentors are involved with a mentee. It is common knowledge that the majority of faculty who have had mentors are more productive in obtaining competitive grants, leading professional organizations, and publishing more books and refereed journal articles. Mentored faculty are also found to have higher job satisfaction.

CONCLUSION

As one realizes the significance that mentoring can have on some individuals, it becomes more readily understood that perhaps there is something to what people say when they describe their mentorship: "I still think about things we used to discuss or I try to think how my mentor would manage a challenge facing me, and it has been 17 years." "I still, after 21 years, use things that I learned from my mentoring experience, and I feel good when something triggers me to remember these 'lessons.' " Siegel (1999) studies the neurology of interpersonal relationships and writes about how we become the people we are through our interpersonal connections. He further elaborates that the mind emerges from the brain and its structures and that functions of the brain are directly shaped by interpersonal relationships. Due to the connection between the brain structure and its function, research has provided new insights into how experience shapes mental processes. So there is more evidence that having a mentor or mentors has a significant impact on humans, and the wisdom and shared learning one can gain from a mentor has a positive influence on our ability to engage in interpersonal relationships throughout life.

Allen and Johnston (2000) cited more than 550 articles published on mentoring in business, education, and nursing. They emphasize there is no one right way to mentor; it depends greatly on multiple variables such as cultural background of the mentor and mentee, geographic distance between the mentor and mentee, the purpose of the mentoring, and the experience of the mentor with mentoring.

The idea of providing mentorships prevails in practice disciplines such as education, business, and nursing. There are opportunities from using best practices in mentoring to:

- develop new models of support for people to succeed;
- maximize creative recruitment and retention strategies for the organization;
- strengthen the profession by producing increased knowledge and theory.

It is becoming more and more evident that teachers and students, supervisors and subordinates, managers and staff, and peers with colleagues are being successful in advancing self, organizational, and professional goals with mentoring. It is important that the various terms used to describe a mentoring process be defined operationally so that individuals have clarity when reading results of research, setting up mentoring programs, and describing their own mentoring experience.

This mentoring experience comprises a skill/content and a psychosocial support component. Most significant, people need to understand the type of relationship that has occurred and how this relationship served the mentor, mentee, organization, and profession. It is realistic for most people to have more than one mentoring experience in their lives and also work with multiple preceptors, coaches, and role models. If someone is fortunate enough to have a long-term mentoring relationship, then this is a classic mentor-mentee relationship. It is in this case that the two individuals willingly spend time together as they share experiences and learn from each other.

Sheehy (1976) calls this partnership that develops over time the *mentor connection* and refers to it as the "secret link to success." Findings that support positive outcomes from the preceptor, coach, and role-model relationships also support success. There is general consensus that individuals who have or have had good mentoring relationships tend to be well balanced with personal and work issues as well as successful in their professional careers. More research identifying best practices in mentoring will serve to accentuate the need for a mentoring culture within and between disciplines.

REFERENCES

Allen, J., & Johnston, K. (1997). Mentoring. *Context, 14*, 15.

Andrews, M., & Wallis, M. (1999). Mentorship in nursing: A literature review. *Journal of Advanced Nursing, 29*, 201–207.

Bell, C. (1998). *Managers as mentors: Building partnerships for learning.* San Francisco: Berrett-Koehler.

Bennetts, C. (2000). The traditional mentor relationship and the well being of creative individuals in school and work. *International Journal of Health Promotion and Education, 38*, 22–27.

Bennis, W. (2004). The seven ages of the leader. *Harvard Business Review, 82*, 46–53.

Boreen, J., & Niday, D. (2003). *Mentoring across boundaries: Helping beginning teachers succeed in challenging situations.* Portland, ME: Stenhouse.

Carew, J. (1998). *The mentor: Fifteen keys to success in sales, business, and life.* New York: Donald Fine Books.

Cross, K. (1981). *Adults as learners.* San Francisco: Jossey-Bass.

Daloz, L. (1999). *Mentor: Guiding the journey of adult learners* (2nd ed.). San Francisco: Jossey-Bass.

Ehrich, L., Tennent, L., & Hansford, B. (2002). Review of mentoring in education: Some lessons for nursing. *Contemporary Nurse, 12*, 253–264.

Erikson, E. (1963). *Childhood and society* (2nd ed.). New York: Norton.

Fenelon, F. (1994). *Les aventures de Telemaque* (P. Riley, trans.). Cambridge: Cambridge University Press. (Original work published 1699.)

Flynn, J. (1997). *The role of the preceptor: A guide for nurse educators and clinicians.* New York: Springer Publishing.

Gay, B. (1994). What is mentoring? *Education and Training, 36*, 4–7.

Gilley, J., & Boughton, N. (1996). *Stop managing, start coaching.* Chicago: Irwin.

Homer. (1946). *The odyssey* (E. V. Rieu, trans.). Harmondsworth, England: Penguin.

Huang, C., & Lynch, J. (1995). *Mentoring: The Tao of giving and receiving wisdom.* New York: Harper.

Jarvis, D. (1992). Improving junior faculty scholarship. In M. Sorcinelli & A. Austin (Eds.), *Developing new and junior faculty.* San Francisco: Jossey-Bass.

Johnson, W., & Huwe, J. (2003). *Getting mentored: In graduate school.* Washington, DC: American Psychological Association.

Joiner, B. (1994). *Fourth generation management: The new business consciousness.* New York: McGraw-Hill.

Kolb, D. (1984). *Experiential learning.* Englewood Cliffs, NJ: Prentice Hall.

Knowles, M. (1984). *Andragogy in action: Applying modern principles of adult learning.* San Francisco: Jossey-Bass.

Kram, K. (1983). Phases of the mentor relationship. *Academy of Management Journal, 26*, 608–625.

Kram, K. (1986). Mentoring in the workplace. In D. Hall (Ed.), *Career development in organizations*. San Francisco: Jossey-Bass.

Lee, L. (2000). Motivation, mentoring, and empowerment aren't just management jargon—they're resources you use every day. *Nursing Management, 10*, 25–28.

Levinson, D., Darrow, E., Klein, M., Levinson, M., & McKee, B. (1978). *The seasons of a man's life*. New York: Knopf.

Luna, G., & Cullen, D. (1996). *Empowering the faculty: Mentoring redirected and renewed*. Washington, DC: George Washington University Press.

McWeeny, M. (2002). The changing mosaic of mentoring. *Creative Nursing Journal, 3*, 3–4.

Miller, A. (2002). *Mentoring students and young people*. Sterling, VA: Stylus Publishing.

Murray, M. (2001). *Beyond the myths and magic of mentoring: How to facilitate an effective mentoring process* (2nd ed.). San Francisco: Jossey-Bass.

National Commission on Teaching in America's Future. Report. (2003). Washington, DC.

Peluchete, J., & Jeanquart, S. (2000). Professionals' use of different mentor sources at various career stages: Implications for career success. *Journal of Social Psychology, 140*, 549–564.

Pollock, R. (1995). A test of conceptual models depicting the developmental course of informal mentor-protégé relationships in the work place. *Journal of Vocational Behavior, 46*, 144–162.

Restifo, V., & Yoder, L. (2004). Partnership: Making the most of mentoring. *Nursing Spectrum, 8*, 16–19.

Roberts, A. (2000). Mentoring revisited: A phenomenological reading of the literature. *Mentoring and Tutoring, 8*, 145–170.

Rymer, J. (2002). "Only connect": Transforming ourselves and our discipline through co-mentoring. *Journal of Business Communication, 39*, 342–364.

Schweibert, V. (2000). *Mentoring: Creating connected, empowered relationships*. Alexandria, VA: American Counseling Association.

Shea, G. (1997). *Mentoring: How to develop successful mentor behaviors*. Menlo Park, CA: Crisp Learning.

Shea, G. (1999). *Making the most of being mentored*. Menlo Park, CA: Crisp Learning.

Sheehy, G. (1976). The mentor connection and the secret link in the successful woman's life. *New York Magazine, 8*, 33–39.

Siegal, D. (1999). *The developing mind: How relationships and the brain interact to shape who we are*. New York: Guilford Press.

Simon, S., & Eby, L. (2003). A typology of negative mentoring experiences: A multidimensional scaling study. *Human Relations, 56*, 1083–1106.

Sinetar, M. (1998). *The mentor's spirit: Life lessons on leadership and the art of encouragement*. New York: St. Martin's Press.

Sue, D. (1981). *Counseling the culturally different*. New York: Wiley.

Weil, V. (2001). Mentoring: Some ethical considerations. *Science and Engineering Ethics, 7*, 471–482.

Wickman, F., & Sjodin, T. (1996). *Mentoring: The most obvious yet overlooked key to achieving more in life than you ever dreamed possible.* New York: McGraw-Hill.

Wilson, J., & Elman, N. (1990). Organizational benefits of mentoring. *Academy of Management Executive, 4*, 88–94.

Zey, M. (1990). *The mentor connection: Strategic alliance in corporate life.* New Brunswick, NJ: Transaction Publications.

CHAPTER 2

Vision of the Mentoring Culture in Nursing

Nursing needs to develop a mentoring culture, that is, all nurses should experience being in a collaborative network that fosters partnering with others. Most nurses today receive precepting during their orientation to a clinical position or coaching for a special project or promotion they are preparing for, or perhaps they look up to someone as a role model who inspires them. But most do not have experience in a classic mentoring dyad or group. The majority of individuals who have had mentoring are doctorally prepared nurses with their dissertation chair, along with some fortunate middle managers in service who may be mentored by their senior nurse administrators. With the new mentoring models such as peer and multiple mentoring, every nurse could benefit from being in a mentoring culture. This culture needs to permeate the nursing workforce so that there is a broader impact not only on individual nurses desiring mentoring but also the organization and the nursing profession. Due to the nature of this emerging workforce with 20-year-olds it is even more critical to mentor effectively by leading individuals to self-empower themselves and increase their self-confidence so they can become effective leaders (Allen, 1998).

DEVELOPING A MENTORING CULTURE

Stewart and Krueger (1996) conducted a concept analysis of mentoring in nursing and suggest its strongest relationship is as a "teaching–learning process for the socialization of nurse scholars and scientists and the proliferation of a body of professional knowledge" (p. 318). Results of this investigation regarding the state of classical mentoring in nursing reflect what is happening in academia. Byrne and Keefe (2002) offer an excellent synopsis of the impact of mentoring on nursing research. Research appears to be the only setting in which long-term mentoring relationships are occurring.

Probably due to the nursing shortage, there is also more interest than ever before in mentoring or guiding students, individuals interested in nursing, and nurses. So what does this mean? Why is it that people are willing to reach out and encourage more individuals to enter the nursing profession? Any nurse would say that it is because nurses are able to make a difference, and if there were to be enough nurses, each nurse could finish the day feeling he or she completed what was planned and made a difference with his or her nursing interventions.

This chapter describes the visions nurses have regarding the development of a mentoring culture so that our profession will be successful in accomplishing its purpose. Nurses need to broaden their connections with others so that each nurse is introduced to the multiple benefits of being networked. It would be advantageous to begin getting involved with this mentoring spirit early in one's career. For example, student nurses could be mentees in their initial academic training with a faculty, clinical nurse, or someone in the university setting, or possibly be mentors for first-year students or someone interested in gaining the kind of experience and knowledge that student mentors can offer. It is known that nurses who have been mentors tend to mentor others (Vance & Olson, 1998; Yoder, 1990). Davidhizar (1988), Roche (1979), and Fagan and Fagan (1983) have found that nurses who have been successfully mentored are more likely to mentor others when compared to those with little or no mentoring experience.

Nurse clinicians can mentor each other as well as new graduates and students, faculty can mentor graduate students regarding their advanced role and in the area of expanding evidence-based practice, and doctoral students can receive mentoring regarding their research. Nurse executives can mentor managers, and managers can mentor staff, and so it goes. Depending on where a nurse is in his or her career, he or she can be a mentor, mentee, or both, and can be in a classic mentoring dyad, a peer network, or multiple mentoring relationships. The majority of nurses think of mentoring as a mechanism for career advancement. Nurses need to think about expanding this view to encompass a broader vision that benefits more than their career. Mentoring can greatly benefit the profession by expanding nursing knowledge and science. Just as Stewart and Krueger (1996) identified in their concept analysis of mentoring that classic mentoring is "a teaching-learning process for the socialization of nurse scholars and scientists and the proliferation of a body of professional knowledge," other types of mentoring are teaching-learning processes by which nurses can be socialized and add findings from evidence-based practice to the body of professional nursing knowledge. This means that more evidence-based practice and study of how nursing influences patient care needs to be conducted on a daily basis where nurses are practicing.

Clinical nurse specialists and the new clinical nurse leader role may allow a mentoring staff to expand the nursing science base in everyday work with patients. Just as a bench scientist works in his or her discipline, nurses need to use their patient assignments as a base for their research. Similarly, every staff nurse has a responsibility to assess, plan, implement, and evaluate the highest-quality care for patients. By facilitating a mentoring culture, nurses can work smarter and not harder by using every individual at the work setting in a way that maximizes this person's abilities. A vision of the mentoring culture in nursing holds exceptional promise for nurses, the profession, the organizations that employ nurses, and, most significant, patients. Additionally, if all nurses develop their mentoring skills, they can be more effective leaders in every health care delivery setting and have more influence in generating positive patient outcomes in health care (Evans & Lang, 2004).

Indicators of a mentoring culture include

- accountability;
- alignment;
- demand;
- infrastructure;
- a common mentoring vocabulary;
- multiple venues;
- reward;
- role modeling;
- safety net;
- training and education (Zachary, 2000).

Zachary (2002) says that an organization that values mentoring has to accept it within its culture. It cannot be considered an add-on. It must be linked with the organization's values and stated in the mission and philosophy. The infrastructure must be supported by human and financial resources. There must be dedicated time spent on training, mentor coaching, and administration of the mentorship. Nurses who are leaders will be accountable for mentoring those who follow them and also their peers. They will be reimbursed for their contributions. Mission statements and philosophies for universities and health care agencies encompass values that are congruent with fostering mentoring in their organizations. Organizational structure and the culture of institutions reflect the milieu of the infrastructure. Nurse administrators can role-model strategies for staff to best support mentoring in their organizations.

Everyone can visualize a specific department, unit, or even health care agency that was especially welcoming and nurturing at some point in her or his career. Likewise, one can appreciate the role models who have assisted in shaping one's career direction and status—the special teacher or staff nurse who took the time to show or explain something one more time. By promoting more recognition of good experiences and role models as Hudacek does in her books, *Making a Difference: Stories From the Point of Care* (2005) and *A Daybook for Nurses: Making a Difference Each Day* (2004), a culture of mentoring can be advanced in nursing. The profession could decide to foster mentoring in a more comprehensive fashion if each nurse became involved in coaching, precepting, or mentoring peers and less experienced colleagues. By establishing mentoring teams, nurses can foster more comprehensive networks and develop best practices in mentoring, as well as socializing nurses to participate in expanding the profession to be a science (Fitzpatrick & Abraham, 1987).

BEST PRACTICES IN MENTORING IN NURSING

The following definition of *mentoring* emerges from the literature on descriptions of mentoring:

> Mentoring in nursing encompasses a guided experience, formally or informally assigned, over a mutually agreed-on period, that empowers the mentor and mentee to develop personally and professionally within the auspices of a caring, collaborative, culturally competent, and respectful environment.

Evidence-based practice in mentoring in nursing can support each component of this definition.

A Guided Experience

Mentor is the term used when discussing mentoring in nursing and is often used interchangeably with *preceptor, coach, assessor, teacher/supervisor*, and *adviser*. Stewart and Krueger (1996) distinguish the separate processes of precepting, coaching, assessing, teaching/supervising, and advising. A *preceptor* is assigned for working alongside and evaluating new employees, a *coach* gives skill training tips on a regular basis, an *assessor* evaluates the employee's performance, the *teacher/supervisor* facilitates new opportunities to increase the person's knowledge and experiential base and acts as a resource, and the *adviser* suggests specific strategies to obtain a degree or advance one's career. In England, *mentor* is identified as being synonymous with *preceptor, supervisor,* and *assessor* (Andrews & Wallis, 1999). So the classic term *mentoring* is loosely used in the nursing profession, and it includes each of these roles being manifested by one experienced individual, over a mutually determined period of time, with a less experienced individual. Stewart and Krueger (1996) studied related concepts of mentoring such as role modeling, sponsoring, precepting, peer strategizing, collaborating, and coaching. Table 2.1 compares and contrasts the definition of these terms during the 1990s and in 2006.

There has been some change in the perception of mentoring and its related roles over the past decade in that co-mentoring and multiple mentoring have greatly increased. There is a great deal of research on the increase in mentoring in the purest sense in doctoral education. Precepting remains the most frequently cited aspect of "mentoring" for nurses today, and it involves assigned relationships with students or new orienting nurses and experienced nurses in a time-limited and evaluation-oriented experience.

Formal Versus Informal Assignments: Stages of the Mentoring Process

Mentoring is considered best when it occurs spontaneously (or is unassigned) between two people (Restifo & Yoder, 2004). There is more informal matching that occurs, and sometimes this mentoring does not continue over an extended period of time. Most nurses have assigned precepting experiences for their orientation to a new unit. Some may ask the preceptor to be their mentor when their orientation comes to a close. Still others network with peers and mentor each other during orientation or a specific course. Andrews and Wallis (1999) suggest that mentoring occurs throughout a person's career, and sometime we are the mentor and other times the mentee. Mentoring occurs at all levels of nursing, is formal or informal, and the mentor can be someone with less experience or education than the mentee if the mentee-mentor relationship allows. There is no one mentoring framework in nursing. There are multiple models that delineate stages of the process for the mentor and mentee. They discuss the importance of nursing students and new graduates learning in classrooms and alongside mentors in clinical practice. They talk about the multiple terms used synonymously with *mentor* such as *preceptor, assessor,* and *supervisor.*

There are no standard stages of mentoring in nursing. Kram's stages (1983) of a mentoring relationship are standard in education. Bower (2000a)

TABLE 2.1   Comparison of Mentoring Roles in 1990s and 2006

Up to 1995	1995–2006
Role Model	
No personal relationship need exist. One person internalizes another's behaviors or standards, which then become her or his own (Stewart & Krueger, 1996).	Often no personal relationship exists. Frequently nurses have several role models for adapting behaviors and strategies that assist with professional and personal growth. *Shadowing* is synonymous with *role modeling.*
Sponsor	
Often money is pledged; a group finds an appropriate reference group for an individual or group of individuals (Stewart & Krueger, 1996).	Term not used in nursing
Preceptor	
A pairing of an experienced employee and new employee for purposes of orienting the new employee. This is an assigned pairing for a limited amount of time, generally for 2 to 4 weeks (Stewart & Krueger, 1996).	An experienced staff nurse (Benner, 1984) is paired with a less experienced nurse, new graduate, or student to orient to a position. Certified nurse practitioners with 2 to 4 years of experience can precept graduate students studying to become nurse practitioners. The preceptor receives credit for recertification for precepting.
Peer Strategizer/Co-Mentor	
People of similar age and experience engage in trading information, guidance, and other assistance to improve at least one of the peer's situations (Stewart & Krueger, 1996).	Peer colleagues network to assist each other. Each individual in the peer network receives beneficial outcomes from this sharing of information and resources.
Coach	
A training technique used over an individual's employment span by management and generally on a day-to-day basis (Stewart & Krueger, 1996).	The process of coaching or helping an individual to use his or her maximum potential has become more respected and viewed as very beneficial for new employees. It is a common process of mentoring nurse managers and administrators.
Multiple Mentoring	
This allows individuals to network and be mentored by several people simultaneously. There is vertical and horizontal mentoring occurring whereby mentees mentor mentors, and each individual does both roles with multiple people at any one time. This process began to evolve in the 1990s.	This simultaneous mentoring network is extremely common today in nursing academia and service.

presents a Mentor Relationship Model that has three stages incorporating Kram's stages (Initiation, Cultivation, Separation, and Redefinition) that are frequently used in nursing:

1. *Selection Process.*   Generally the mentor chooses the mentee, but there are exceptions when the mentee picks the mentor. Bower feels that due to burnout of nurses, there is more interest in mentoring than ever before. Due to this interest in strengthening the profession, more nurse leaders seem to be mentoring more mentees. During this initial stage of the relationship, it is important for the mentor and mentee to determine if they are compatible, assess their similarities and differences, and determine if they have mutual goals. It is significant that both parties develop trust, and it is fairly easy to see if they are going to be able to work effectively together. Once the selection is made, the following must occur: the mentor agrees to spend a specific amount of time with the mentee; the mentor must be willing to open his or her network of colleagues up to the mentee, the mentor must assess if he or she has the skills to assist the mentee in accomplishing goals, and the mentor must give the mentee access or availability.

2. *Goal-Setting Phase.*   The goals may already be developed by the mentee or the mentee's organization. The mentor may have some guidelines to assist in developing goals, or the two may want to mutually develop the goals. Communication is key for success, and the mentor and mentee must have excellent and frequent communication regarding goal evaluation and progress.

3. *Working Phase.*   Initially the mentor sets up activities and work for the mentee to accomplish. Once this is completed, the mentee may suggest certain ideas for the mentor to respond to. This brings the relationship to more of an exchange, and the mentor and mentee become more of a team and work together to accomplish the established goals. It is crucial that both the mentor and mentee feel comfortable in giving each other feedback. If goals continue to be accomplished and the team works successfully together, then the transition step of the working phase will occur. This is the transition of mentee to colleague status.

Another mentoring process by Fox and Shephard (1998) identified three phases—(1) recognition and development, (2) limited independence, and (3) termination and realignment—that seem similar to Bower's and Kram's. No stages of preceptorships were identified in the literature. However, if the evaluation aspect of a relationship is formal and determines the mentee's fate in a work setting, then the relationship is a preceptorship, not a mentorship.

Bower (2000a) shares examples of her experiences as a mentor and also how she was mentored. Mentoring has been studied in all facets of the profession. It is recommended for use in academia (undergraduate through doctoral levels), clinical settings for all roles (this is generally a preceptorship), political arenas, nursing organizations, and as prenurse matching programs in communities during high school or middle school.

Mutually Agreed-On Duration

As mentoring evolves into other forms besides the classic dyad relationship, it becomes more difficult to identify specified periods of time for the relationship. Most feel the classic mentoring relationship exists at least 5 years, and many say these relationships never really end.

Positive Outcomes Generated for Mentor and Mentee

Mentoring is one of the core competencies that leaders must have (Grossman & Valiga, 2005; Iberre, 2000; Lanser, 2000; Mitchell, 2004; Ross, Wenzel, & Mitlyng, 2002). Mentoring that takes place between an experienced nurse leader and a mentee will generate success for both parties, plus the organization that employs each and the profession of nursing. Outcomes such as improved retention rate of graduate nurses (Almada, Carafoli, Flattery, French, & McNamera, 2004), increased leadership skills for nurses (Grossman, 2005; Nickitas, Keida, Nokes, & Neville, 2004), increased faculty tenure and promotions (Abel, 2004; Snelson et al., 2002), and increased use of resources for academia and health care agency (Kinnaman & Bleich, 2004; Novotny, Donahue, & Bhalla, 2004) are some of the outcomes produced by having a mentoring culture. Partnering continues to be extremely important for institutions of higher educations and health care agencies in order to accomplish goals of finding clinical placements and recruiting new graduates; however, even more outcomes from these partnerships have evolved. Achieving magnet status, research collaboration between academicians and clinicians, cost reduction for both parties, tuition-free courses taught at the health care agency, collaborative grant-writing projects, adjunct teaching positions for clinicians, and sharing of resources are some of the benefits of these practice-education collaborations.

Stewart and Krueger (1996) find in their literature review that outcomes generated by the classic mentor and mentee relationship in the early 1990s included the following:

Progression of one's career
Development of new investigators
Empowerment for mentee
Increased professional knowledge and practice base
Generativity for mentor
Increased numbers of minorities in postbaccalaureate programs
Institutional staff retention
Professional socialization

Over the decade, 1995–2005, the following outcomes of classical mentoring seem apparent, although there are no substantiating data:

- Increased mentoring regarding assisting faculty with developing their research trajectory and obtaining outside funding
- Increased mentoring of nursing faculty and doctoral students regarding research in specific institutions
- Generally increased mentoring for those who are culturally diverse or attempts to provide more role modeling, networking, and shadowing experiences
- Increased partnering between academia and health care agencies for nursing students to work with the agency's experienced nurses
- Increased formal and informal matching of experienced practicing nurses by professional organizations with student nurses and new graduates
- Increased matching of middle and high school students interested in nursing with experienced nurses or a specific group of nurses.
- Recommended for use in academia, clinical settings for all roles, political arenas, nursing organizations, and in communities for those in middle or high school who are interested in nursing.

Bower (2000b), a previous president of Sigma Theta Tau International, writes that succession planning, or a deliberative method of developing the next cadre of leaders, must include mentoring. In her book, *Nurses Taking the Lead* (2000a), Bower shares her perception of how having and being a mentor gives one the "skill of gaining recognition, power, and the ability to influence others" (p. 255), which is the outcome nurses are seeking.

Caring, Culturally Competent, and Respectful Environment

Mentors, like preceptors and coaches, can help to provide a safer, less chaotic, and less frantic environment for nurses to deliver the highest quality of care. Dombeck (1999) says, "A mentor relationship is a gift, it is a profound and humbling process. The gift comes from knowing a person and from being given the privilege of watching him/her in the process of professional development" (p. 2). She identifies the mentor's and mentee's promise to share resources and experiences faithfully as the most valuable part of this relationship. This promise is set in the context of a covenant and is dependent on the capacity to listen not only to mentees' questions but to their souls. She feels faculty in a professional school and clinicians in a professional discipline are roles that require ethical commitment.

MENTORING IN NURSING

Stewart and Krueger (1996) examined 82 research abstracts and articles written between 1977 and 1994. This collection was a randomly chosen sample from the nursing literature in Canada, the United Kingdom, and the United States. They identify six attributes of mentoring using concept analysis:

1. *Mentoring is a teaching and learning strategy.*   Literature to support mentoring as a teaching and learning process is presented, but the authors point out that there is no evidence whether mentoring is an effective teaching and learning format, which mentoring process has the largest impact on learning, or a rationale for how mentoring can facilitate a comprehensive body of nursing knowledge. Fitzpatrick and Abraham (1991) say that mentoring is critical in doctoral education if the teaching-learning objectives involve research and grant-writing skills, as well as other professional scholarly activities. Over the past decade, this concept of mentoring has continued to evolve exponentially in doctoral education. Master's and baccalaureate education programs seem to have less mentoring and more coaching and try to have transition experiences for seniors that match them with a preceptor, not a mentor. Health care agencies foster preceptorship with their experienced employees and new employees. It would be interesting to determine how many of these preceptorships develop into mentorships. Professional organizations recommend that every nurse have a mentor, and some organizations try to match their members with nurses interested in the organization's focus. This is more of a coaching and role-modeling process and is aimed more at career growth. It is not clear which part of the mentoring process seems to benefit the mentee's career or the profession the most.

2. A mentoring relationship has reciprocal roles between the mentor and mentee.   This concept has become more universally accepted for a classically defined mentorship. With the increase in peer and multiple mentoring, it becomes evident that both mentors and mentees benefit from the learning generated from the mentorship.

3. Mentoring assists in advancement of career for both the mentor and mentee.   Although the majority of mentoring relationships concentrate on career development, there is a general move toward increasing efforts of mentoring to include development of the profession. Ardery (1990) proposes that mentors and mentees focus on professional success versus personal success so that knowledge generated from the mentorship can advance nursing theory. This does not seem to have occurred, since research is still dominated by measurements of mentee success with publications, presentations, obtaining grants in their specific area of research, and rate of tenure, promotion, and other gauges of career advancement.

4. There is generally a knowledge differential between the mentor and mentee.   The idea of the mentor being more knowledgeable than the mentee continues to hold true in classically defined mentoring relationships. However, the growth in the number of peer mentoring and multiple mentoring relationships provides some evidence that this concept may be arguable.

5. A classic mentorship consists of a long-term relationship extending over several years.   Mentoring relationships on the average tend to endure. This literature review revealed a range of between 1.5 and 33 years.

6. Mentoring tends to generate resonance.   Mentoring assists participants in developing character and doing higher-quality work.

These six themes seem to be congruent with what is current now, with the added emphasis on mentoring for the profession. There is also no formal evaluation process in a mentoring relationship.

Mentoring in Clinical Settings

There are multiple accounts of supporting new graduates in internships or extended orientations, retooling nurses who have not practiced in awhile, and orienting experienced nurses to new experiences (Morton-Cooper & Palmer, 1993). Nurse managers also need to hone their own career guidance skills to effectively develop staff nurses as employees. Help with getting acclimated to a new job and advancing one's career greatly assists a new nurse's successful transition to an entry-level staff nurse position from student status. Mentoring is necessary to assist the profession with the worldwide nursing shortage because mentoring programs can help decrease attrition in educational programs and also increase recruitment and retention in health care agencies. In a study by Boswell and Wilhoit (2004), nurses ($N = 67$) identified the following three processes as being what they perceived as most responsible for generating high-quality nursing:

- Comprehensive orientation on hiring or transfer to a new unit
- A variety of continuing education programs offered frequently and at the hospital
- Mentoring

Of course, it is possible that a new graduate will be involved in a preceptorship that will progress to being a mentor-mentee relationship. If, after the new graduate satisfies the competency-based objectives at the end of orientation for his or her unit, the preceptor and the new graduate may wish to extend their relationship on a more informal and nonevaluative basis. The relationship could then become a mentorship. Often new graduates also develop a peer mentoring network that is extremely helpful in their transition to staff nurse status. Vance (1999) cites the following behavior exhibited by the graduates often as most instrumental in triggering longer-term mentoring:

- Initiates asking for advice from other nurses
- Demonstrates seriousness about his or her position
- Maintains his or her own identity

It is important to realize that the mentorship will extend beyond the specific job and assist the new nurse in becoming socialized into the professional nurse's role.

Angelini (1995) conducted a qualitative grounded theory study to identify how mentoring influenced the career development of hospital staff nurses. Environment, people, and events were identified as significant to mentoring. Both the staff nurses and manager defined mentoring as broader than just the dyad. The nurses felt that the environment consisted of what the hospital offered them, such as tuition reimbursement, other educational opportunities at the hospital, chances to consult with other nurses, and financial rewards. "People" included both primary and secondary mentors (people who influenced them), with the primary ones being nurse managers and peer staff nurses with whom they interacted frequently and the secondary people being less frequent contacts, such as clinical nurse specialists, nurse educators, family members, and physicians. "Events" included occurrences perceived to be critical to career development, such as clinical patient situations and career incidents (first job, first charge, first transfer, first float). And outside influences involved family, social events, and issues such as the women's movement. Angelini's conclusions include that true mentoring takes on primary importance at the clinical bedside but generally does occur in every aspect of life.

There are studies of students often in their senior year doing their capstone experience that have had a semester-long, assigned "mentor"—literally, a preceptor. Each preceptorship is different and is influenced by multiple variables. Some (Greene & Puetzer, 2002; Grossman, 2005) suggest that the prime time to introduce nurses to a mentor relationship is during the student experience since academia is responsible for preparing nurses for their first role in patient care delivery. Several have published their experiences in providing students with some form of mentoring in a nursing care setting. Grossman (2005) describes a shadowing experience for senior students in a leadership and management rotation in which each student was assigned a leader in a health care agency to shadow over a semester. Findings revealed statistically significant increased leadership development scores after the mentorship. Papp, Markkanen, and von Bonsdorff (2003) reported that student nurses perceived more positive learning environments when nurse educators and staff nurses worked closely together in providing precepted clinical experiences.

Practice learning accounts for about 50% of the prequalifying nursing program in the United Kingdom. Andrews and Wallis (1999) were most interested in determining what teaching-learning strategies best support students. Mentorship is widely relied on to teach the main activities associated with practice skills. Recently nurse educators in the United Kingdom have also applied the mentorship strategy in classroom teaching. Outcomes are not yet available.

The Institute of Nursing Executives in Australia answered the concern of their members by developing a mentoring program to provide professional development and support networks for nurse managers working in rural areas. A pilot program developed in and around Sydney required the managers and mentors to attend a full-day mentoring workshop. There was time set aside for mentors and mentees to form partnerships. Seventy-nine percent of the participants responded to a preworkshop questionnaire asking for their most significant learning needs. They cited learning how to increase their confidence in coaching and stimulating staff as their primary learning need. Managers' evaluations of the program expressed a need for more networking, more structured mentoring, and training to assist them in using technology to keep involved in their newly established mentor-ships and networks. Outcomes of the project included the development of a mentoring listserv and Web site to assist managers (Waters, Clarke, In-gall, & Dean-Jones, 2003).

There are also studies of graduate students being precepted. Research indicates a definitive need for these programs to retain nurses and prepare them adequately for RN and APRN positions. Hayes (1998, 2001) discusses factors that increase self-efficacy as well as mentoring scores for nurse prac-titioner students and points out that nurse practitioner students do better with self-efficacy scores if they can pick their own mentor nurse practi-tioner, particularly if they had a previous relationship with that person. This information is especially helpful for nurse practitioner program direc-tors who may have been making extremely time-consuming assignments of procuring preceptors. Also it is necessary to mentor or precept nurse prac-titioner students regarding other activities that affect patient care but are not involved in direct care, such as research, consultation, counseling, teaching, quality assurance, case management, and health policy develop-ment. A study conducted in the mid-1990s (Thibodeau & Hawkins, 1994) found that many times, nurse practitioner students are not socialized into the multifaceted nurse practitioner role due to the time constraints of nurse practitioners in most practice arenas. It is therefore extremely important for nurse practitioner faculty to role-model and provide seminars, share rele-vant experiences about their own practice, and provide opportunities for their students during the educational period. Often graduate nurse practi-tioners keep in touch with their faculty for advice on negotiating a contract, obtaining malpractice insurance and affiliation privileges, and just talking about day-to-day practice concerns. The National Organization of Nurse Practitioner Faculty (NONPF) has a Web site, www.nonpf.org, with re-sources for mentoring nurse practitioner students as well as graduates.

Due to low staffing, heavy acuity, and lack of resources, there is an in-tense need for appropriate supervision and mentorship of nursing students. The School of Nursing at the University of Nottingham, England, developed a student peer support supervision program in which senior students su-pervise and support junior students in their clinical rotations under the mentorship of a clinical nurse. Three themes were identified after analyzing results of a questionnaire given to 31 seniors and 27 juniors:

1. Preparation for clinical assignment
2. Support and feedback regarding their performance
3. Personal and professional development

This program was evaluated overwhelmingly positively by both groups of students. Seniors commented on improving their teaching and mentoring skills, and juniors felt the program helped to decrease their anxiety and provide needed support (Aston & Molassiotis, 2003).

Mentoring in the Classroom

Andrews and Roberts (2003) say mentoring is important in the classroom as well as in clinical rotations. Nurse educators need to mentor their students. Nurse educators can assist students to be academically successful. Shelton (2003) found a significant relationship between faculty support and student retention and success. It is evident that undergraduate faculty will not be able to have a classic mentoring relationship with every student. Rather, faculty can mentor in groups, assist students in finding a preceptor in their clinical rotation, and advise students in groups as well as individually as the situation arises and also in anticipation of specific events. Graduate faculty need to mentor their students in the more traditional way or find a preceptor who will be working with the graduate student and could serve as a mentor. Doctoral students should have a classic mentor in order to be successful with their research. Nursing faculty engaged in research are the best mentors for students. These students need to develop grantsmanship and research skills, and become connected to the other researchers in their chosen area of study (Byrne & Keefe, 2002). Faculty mentors must assist with increasing self-esteem, be available for support and advice, be a good role model by teaching by example, try to connect students to opportunities for new experiences, try to support passion and vision, and give career advice.

On graduation, most new graduates are assigned to a preceptor, and if they have had experience with some form of mentoring, they will most likely maximize their experience as a preceptee. The preceptee will also know the advantages of trying to continue a supportive relationship with the preceptor after orientation ends. Simultaneously, new graduates will be aware of the advantages of keeping their relationship with someone from their school of nursing or will begin to shape a new relationship with someone at their employing agency. New graduates can foster the mentoring culture in their work setting by demonstrating behavior that recognizes the importance of encouraging and supporting others.

Multiple mentoring encourages maximal growth and probably increases outcomes at the work or school setting. This win-win combination is the future of a more collaborative working nurse force. Turning from a task orientation to more of a relationship paradigm will allow for improved work production and assist the nurse in delegating and seeing patients differently.

There have been several courses offered for undergraduate nursing students that involved long-term mentoring after the official completion of the semester (Inouye, 1995; Morrison-Beady, Aronowitz, Dyne, & Mkandawire, 2001; Perry, 1997). Byrne and Keefe (2002) recommend that more mentoring in research be performed with undergraduate and master's students. They believe that more mentored research will occur where there are faculty funded by the National Institutes of Health (NIH) who need research assistants and at universities with academic health centers conducting clinical research.

Research Mentoring of Doctoral Students

Byrne and Keefe (2002) relate that the major focus of classic mentoring in nursing has shifted to mentoring nurse researchers. They provide descriptions of strategies for setting up research mentorships and describe five research mentoring models:

1. Traditional one-on-one mentor to mentee
2. A team of mentors working with one mentee
3. Peer-to-peer mentors
4. One mentor and a group of mentees
5. Initial traditional mentor to mentee, which then becomes a collegial peer relationship

There is a critical need for development of nurse researchers and only a limited number of institutions are equipped to prepare scholars in an accelerated manner. Providing mentoring throughout undergraduate and graduate education by funded faculty researchers is advocated. Accelerated NIH-funded schools with research-intensive tracks that link baccalaureate through doctoral education right to postdoctoral training are needed in order to prepare nurse research academicians. Perhaps a program similar to the 7-year premedical and medical school programs could be a model for nurses to build a similar prenursing and nurse doctoral program.

Research Mentoring of Faculty

Records and Emerson (2003) share a comprehensive research skill development mentoring model they developed for new faculty at their institution that includes assigning the mentee to two seasoned faculty researchers. The researchers assist in developing annual goals over a 6-year time span, such as submitting two manuscripts, presenting at one conference, and obtaining at least one potential consultant who can assist them with their research funding the first year. The mentors schedule meetings along the 6-year time line. Mentors read the new faculty member's dissertation and assist the person in developing manuscript ideas, select the top researchers in the mentee's field who are in the geographical area, assist with grant writing, suggest methods for networking with them and ways to access research participants and funding, and even give advice concerning how to gracefully decline offers of assistance from those who do not facilitate progress. With the nursing faculty shortage, it would seem prudent for all schools of nursing to engage in a similar mentoring program for new faculty.

Schmitt (1999) echoes in a *Research in Nursing and Health* editorial what other experienced nurse researchers are saying: "Helping the next generation envision who they are individually and collectively is central" (p. 1) to what retiring nurse academicians should be doing. Schmitt (1998) also offers ideas regarding how mentors can assist future nurse scholars. Baggs (1998) sets out strategies for faculty groups to assist each other in editing manuscripts.

Byrne and Keefe (2002) reviewed the literature on research mentoring of faculty. They describe one study of 305 doctorally prepared female faculty working in graduate programs in the United States. Only 56% of the participants reported having had mentorships; however, having a mentorship did not correlate highly with funded research. The actual productivity of scholarship was higher for both the mentee and mentor than for faculty who were not in a mentorship. Targeted mentoring relationships were started at the University of Louisville, which connected faculty with productive researchers outside the institution (Mundt, 2001). This strategy did result in increased productivity and funding. Carlson and Rotondo (2001) cite that tenured full professors who are committed to succession planning for the profession are able to do the most mentoring. If they are not involved in funded research, they will be unable to properly mentor new faculty with their scholarship needs. This is where the nonfunded research faculty could mentor the junior faculty for service and teaching but acquire assistance from outside the institution for research mentoring.

Gray and Armstrong (2003) cite the need for new training and nurturing of young research faculty and especially target the need for nurse researchers. They offer suggestions for developing new programs to train and mentor a critical mass of nurse academics so they will be able to assume leadership. They recommend the Quebec Model of Support Health Research

Networks, which fosters more cross-discipline training and mentoring of nurses and other members of the health team.

INTERNATIONAL MENTORING

Byrne and Keefe (2002) report on the multiple partnerships that are occurring across boundaries regarding common patient care issues. There is much disparity between the programs regarding resources for research, so there has emerged a great need for mentoring. They report several examples of collaborations between the University of Pennsylvania School of Nursing and the Henrietta Szold Hadassah/Hebrew University in Israel related to maternal-child health (Medoff-Cooper & Dekeyser, 1998), Columbia University School of Nursing with Göthenburg University in Sweden related to pediatric home care (Byrne, 1998; Lundblad, Byrne, & Hellstrom, 2001), and Pace University School of Nursing with the University of Utrecht in the Netherlands related to management self-efficacy in diabetes mellitus (Shortridge-Baggett & van der Bijl, 1996). With the increased technology today, mentors can communicate with mentees or coach a group of faculty in another country easily. The classic mentoring method does not tend to be successful due to the distance and multiple needs of many of the mentees. The multiple mentoring and peer mentoring models seem as if they will be most effective. There is an abundance of advantages from mentoring and conducting international research (Brathwaite, 2002).

CULTURALLY COMPETENT MENTORING

Martin, Yarbrough, and Alfred (2003) conducted a study of associate and baccalaureate nursing degree graduates in Texas ($N = 1,450$) with the Nurses Professional Value Scale (NPVS) to measure their professional values. Their findings revealed no difference in total score; however, the associate degree graduates did significantly better than baccalaureate graduates on five of the scales: client privacy, accountability for nursing action, acceptance of responsibility and seeks consultation when appropriate, participation in efforts to improve standards of nursing, and collaboration with other team members to meet health needs of public. Their findings suggest the need for increased mentoring regarding professional values, especially with diverse student populations.

The fact that there is a separate component of this chapter on multicultural competence speaks to the lack of integration of cultural competency in the majority of mentoring models. Most preceptors are not of the same culture as their preceptee, so it is of utmost importance to have preceptors trained in cultural competency. Actually, all nurses and health care workers should be trained, and there should be multiple strategies by which heightened awareness could be achieved (Morales-Mann & Higuchi, 1995). Some mentors and mentees may be from the same culture but have very different levels of cultural sensitivity. Coffman, Shellman, and Bernal (2004) suggest that nurses lack cultural self-efficacy, information, and experience with culturally diverse groups. Cultural stereotypes for Asian Americans, Hispanic Americans, and African Americans need to be dispersed, and perhaps doing role plays of some of these issues would serve to increase awareness among preceptors so they do not show prejudice to their preceptees.

EXAMPLES OF DEVELOPING MENTORING EXPERIENCE IN NURSING

The 2004 American Academy of Nursing Annual Conference brochure for Leadership for Health Building on the Past, Creating the Future featured an anonymous quotation: "Good leaders do not always lead; they teach others to lead." This is the essence of what a good leader does when mentoring others. Mentoring has become so important that the U.S. Public Health Service (PHS) Nursing Department directed each category's Professional Advisory Committee (PAC) to develop mentoring programs. Hence, a PHS nurse mentoring directory evolved that consists of volunteer civil servants and commissioned officer nurses who are willing to mentor. The directory says that mentors provide information on duty assignments, details, career advancement, the agencies within which they serve, licensure, and uniform etiquette.

The Oncology Nursing Job Shadowing/Mentoring Program Tool Kit can be obtained from the Oncology Nurses Association. It has several goals, including increasing awareness in oncology nursing careers to students and RNs, assisting nursing schools to help students understand oncology nursing, and assisting mentors in mentoring nurses and students interested in oncology nursing. The National Mentoring Network based in the United Kingdom, which can be accessed at www.mentors.ca or www.peer.ca, provides information on mentoring definitions, gender issues in mentoring, mentoring as a driver for change, finding a mentor, and evaluating mentoring.

Just about every professional journal has recently published more than one article a year on mentoring. Table 2.2 indicates some selected examples

TABLE 2.2   Selected Examples of Mentoring Articles, 2003

Journals & Author	Title
Imprint (Roman, 2003)	"The Importance of Mentoring in the Transition from Student to Nurse"
Reflections in Nursing Leadership (Medoff-Cooper, 2003)	"Advancing Nursing Through Mentoring"
Journal of Nursing Education (Childs, 2003)	"Mentoring Youth: A Service-Learning Course within a College of Nursing"
Journal of Professional Nursing (Byrne, 2003)	"A Mentored Experience (K01) in Maternal-Infant Research"
Nursing in Focus (Brennan, 2003)	"Mentoring and the Mentor Match Program"
Journal of School Nursing (Houghton, 2003)	"A Mentoring Program for New School Nurses"

for the year 2003. Since the mid-1990s, there have been multiple articles explaining mentoring programs, with RNs or nursing students being paired with a more experienced person to achieve a specific goal—usually to orient or educate the less experienced person to a new position or, in some instances, to the profession of nursing. What generally is not as clear is what the authors mean by mentoring. Most of the articles listed in Table 2.2 identify role modeling/shadowing, precepting, and coaching rather than the classic mentoring relationship even though they use the term *mentor* in their title.

It would seem that any introduction to receiving support from an experienced individual is a positive experience for the nurse or student. These accounts will assist in developing a mentoring culture in the profession. Observing nurse leaders helps new nurses cultivate new skills in leadership, management, and clinical practice.

CONCLUSION

There is the beginning of a mentoring culture in the nursing profession, as evidenced by accounts in the literature of successful mentoring in the clinical arena with nurses, advanced practice nurses, managers, and students, as well as in the classroom. Mentoring is evolving to more of a multiple mentor process for most nurses except for doctoral students and junior faculty. It is paramount that nurses use best practices in mentoring regarding the various components of the process:

- A guided but nonevaluated experience
- Formal versus informal assignment/stages of relationship
- Mutually agreed-on duration
- Positive outcomes generated for mentor and mentee
- Caring, culturally competent, respectful environment

There is more awareness of the need for continued mentoring with international research initiatives. Benefits from these partnerships will gain recognition for the mentor, mentee, the involved organizations, and the profession.

Mentoring in nursing encompasses a guided experience, whether it is formally or informally assigned over a mutually agreed-on period, that empowers the mentor and mentee to develop personally and professionally within the auspices of a caring, collaborative, culturally competent, and respectful environment. Evidence-based practice in mentoring in nursing can support each component of this definition.

REFERENCES

Abel, E. (2004). Faculty response to faculty-nurse mentoring. *Journal of Holistic Nursing, 22*, 186–188.

Allen, D. (1998). How many nurses become leaders: Perception and beliefs about leadership development. *Journal of Nursing Administration, 28*, 15–20.

Almada, P., Carafoli, K., Flattery, J., French, D., & McNamera, M. (2004). Improving the retention rate of newly graduated nurses. *Journal for Nurses in Staff Development, 20*, 268–273.

Andrews, M., & Roberts, D. (2003). Supporting student nurses learning in and through clinical practice: The role of the clinical guide. *Nurse Education Today, 23*, 474–481.

Andrews, M., & Wallis, M. (1999). Mentorship in nursing: A literature review. *Journal of Advanced Nursing, 29*, 201–207.

Angelini, D. (1995). Mentoring in the career development of hospital staff nurses: Models and strategies. *Journal of Professional Nursing, 11*, 89–97.

Ardery, G. (1990). Mentors and protégés: From ideology to knowledge. In J. McCloskey & H. Grace (Eds.), *Current issues in nursing* (pp. 58–63). St. Louis: Mosby.

Aston, L., & Molassiotis, A. (2003). Supervising and supporting student nurses in clinical placements: The peer support initiative. *Nurse Education Today, 23*, 202–210.

Baggs, J. (1998) Please join our scholarly group: Valuing the manuscript review process. *Research in Nursing and Health, 21*,101–102.

Benner, P. (1984). *From novice to expert: Excellence and power in clinical nursing practice.* Menlo Park, CA: Addison-Wesley.

Boswell, S., & Wilhoit, K. (2004). New nurses' perceptions of nursing practice and quality patient care. *Journal of Nursing Care Quality, 19,* 76–81.

Bower, F. (2000a). *Nurses taking the lead: Personal qualities of effective leadership.* Philadelphia: Saunders.

Bower, F. (2000b). Succession planning: A strategy for taking charge. *Nursing Leadership Forum, 4,* 110–114.

Braitwaite, D. (2002). Mentoring relationships while conducting international research. *Multicultural Nursing Health, 8,* 36–41.

Brennan, P. (2003). Mentoring and the Mentor Match Program. *Nursing in Focus, 4,* 6.

Byrne, M. W. (1998). Productive international faculty exchange: Columbia University to Gothenburg University example. *Journal of Advanced Nursing, 27,* 1296–1304.

Byrne, M. W. (2003). A mentored experience (KO1) in maternal-infant research. *Journal of Professional Nursing, 19,* 66–75.

Byrne, M., & Keefe, M. (2002). Building research competence in nursing through mentoring. *Journal of Nursing Scholarship, 34,* 391–396.

Carlson, D., & Rotondo, C. (2001). Building research competence in nursing through mentoring. *Advanced Nursing, 27,* 1296–1304.

Childs, J., Sepples, S., & Moody, K. (2003). Educational innovations: Mentoring youth: A service-learning course within a college of nursing. *Journal of Nursing Education, 42,* 182–185.

Coffman, M., Shellman, J., & Bernal, H. (2004). An integrative review of American nurses' perceived cultural self-efficacy. *Journal of Nursing Scholarship, 36,* 180–185.

Davidhizar, R. (1988). Mentoring in doctoral education. *Journal of Advanced Nursing, 13,* 775–781.

Dombeck, M. (1999). The mentor relationship. *Research in Nursing and Health, 22,* 1–2.

Evans, L., & Lang, N. (Eds.). (2004). *Academic nursing practice: Helping to shape the future of healthcare.* New York: Springer Publishing.

Fagan, M., & Fagan, P. (1983). Mentoring among nurses. *Nursing and Health Care, 4,* 77–82.

Fitzpatrick, J., & Abraham, I. (1987). Toward the socialization of scholars and scientists. *Nurse Educator, 12,* 23–25.

Fox, S., & Shephard, T. (1998). The essence of mentoring. *Journal of Neuroscience Nursing, 30,* 1–3.

Gray, J., & Armstrong, P. (2003). Academic health leadership: Looking to the future. *Clinical Investigational Medicine, 26,* 315–326.

Greene, M., & Puetzer, M. (2002). The value of mentoring: A strategic approach to retention and recruitment. *Journal of Nursing Care Quality, 17,* 63–70.

Grossman, S. (2005). Developing leadership through shadowing a leader care. In H. Feldman & M. Greenberg (Eds.), *Educating for leadership (C* pp. 266–278). New York: Springer Publishing.

Grossman, S., & Valiga, T. (2005). *The new leadership challenge: Creating the future of nursing* (2nd ed.). Philadelphia: F. A. Davis.

Hayes, E. (1998). Mentoring and nurse practitioner student self-efficacy. *Western Journal of Nursing Research, 20*, 521–535.

Hayes, E. (2001). Factors that facilitate or hinder mentoring in the nurse practitioner preceptor/student relationship. *Clinical Excellence for Nurse Practitioners, 5*, 111–118.

Houghton, C. (2003). A mentoring program for new school nurses. *Journal of School Nursing, 19*, 24–29.

Hudacek, S. (Ed.). (2005). *Making a difference: Stories from the point of care*. Indianapolis, IN: Sigma Theta Tau International.

Hudacek, S. (2004). *A daybook for nurses: Making a difference each day*. Indianapolis, IN: Center Nursing Press.

Iberre, H. (2000). Making partner: A mentor's guide to the psychological journey. *Harvard Business Review, 78*, 148–149.

Inouye, J. (1995). A research development program for minority honors students. *Journal of Nursing Education, 34*, 268–271.

Kinnaman, M., & Bleich, M. (2004). Collaboration: Aligning resources to create and sustain partnerships. *Journal of Professional Nursing, 20*, 310–322.

Kram, K. (1983). Phases of the mentor relationship. *Academy of Management Journal, 26*, 608–625.

Lanser, E. (2000). Reaping the benefits of mentorship. *Healthcare Executive, 15*, 19–23.

Lundblad, B., Byrne, M., & Hellstrom, A. (2001). Continuing nursing care needs of children at time of discharge from one regional medical center in Sweden. *Journal of Pediatric Nursing, 16*, 73–78.

Martin, P., Yarbrough, S., & Alfred, D. (2003). Professional values held by baccalaureate and associate degree nursing students. *Journal of Nursing Scholarship, 35*, 291–296.

Medoff-Cooper, B. (2003). Advancing nursing through mentoring. *Reflections on Nursing Leadership, 29*, 30.

Medoff-Cooper, B., & Dekeyser, F. (1998). Developing a research mentoring partnership in Israel. *Journal of Obstetric, Gynecologic, and Neonatal Nursing, 27*, 197–202.

Mitchell, G. (2004). The mentoring of nurses: Possibilities for times of transition. *Nursing Science Quarterly, 17*, 317–324.

Morton-Cooper, A., & Palmer, A. (1993). *Mentorship and preceptorship: A guide to support roles in clinical practice*. London: Blackwell Science.

Morales-Mann, E., & Higuchi, K. (1995). Trans-cultural mentoring: An experience in perspective transformation. *Journal of Nursing Education, 34*, 272–277.

owitz, T., Dyne, J., & Mkandawire, L. (2001). Mentoring faculty in funded research: A win-win scenario. *Journal of* , 17, 291–296.

.n external mentor program: Stimulus for faculty research nal of Professional Nursing, 17, 40–45.

Nokes, K., & Neville, S. (2004). Nurturing nursing future xecutive partnerships. *Nursing Economics, 22,* 258–263.

.ue, M., & Bhalla, B. (2004). The clinical partnership as strate- *Journal of Professional Nursing, 20,* 216–221.

Papp, T., Markkanen, M., & von Bonsdorff, M. (2003). Clinical environment as a learning environment: Student nurses' perceptions concerning clinical learning experiences. *Nurse Education Today, 23,* 262–268.

Perry, L. (1997). The bridge program: An overview. *Association of Black Nursing Faculty Journal, 8,* 4–7.

Records, K., & Emerson, R. (2003). Mentoring for research skill development. *Journal of Nursing Education, 42,* 553–557.

Restifo, V., & Yoder, L. (2004). Partnership: Making the most of mentoring. *Nursing Spectrum, 8,* 16–19.

Roche, G. (1979). Much ado about mentoring. *Harvard Business Review, 57,* 14–28.

Roman, M. (2003). The importance of mentoring in the transition from student to nurse. *Imprint, 50,* 50–53.

Ross, A., Wenzel, F., & Mitlyng, J. (2002). *Leadership for the future: Core competencies in health care.* Chicago: Health Administration Press.

Schmitt, M. (1998). Assuring the production of scholars who will continue to build nursing knowledge into the new millennium. *Research in Nursing and Health, 21,* 187–188.

Schmitt, M. (1999). Editorial on mentoring. *Research in Nursing and Health, 22,* 1–2.

Shelton, E. (2003). Faculty support and student retention. *Journal of Nursing Education, 42,* 68–76.

Shortridge-Baggett, L., & van der Bijl, J. (1996). International collaborative research on managing self-efficacy in diabetes mellitus. *Journal of New York State Nurses Association, 3,* 9–14.

Snelson, C., Martsolf, D., Dieckman, B., Anaya, E., Cartehine, K., Miller, B., et al. (2002). Caring as a theoretical perspective for a nursing faulty mentoring program: Mentoring program for new faculty. *Nursing Education Today, 22,* 654–660.

Stewart, B., & Krueger, L. (1996). An evolutionary concept analysis of mentoring in nursing. *Journal of Professional Nursing, 12,* 311–321.

Stone, F. (1999). *Coaching, counseling, and mentoring: How to choose and use the right technique to boost employee performance.* New York: American Management Association.

Thibodeau, J., & Hawkins, J. (1994). Moving toward a nursing model in advanced practice. *Western Journal of Nursing Research, 16,* 205–218.

Waters, D., Clarke, M., Ingall, A., & Dean-Jones, M. (2003). Evaluation of a pilot mentoring program for nurse managers. *Journal of Advanced Nursing, 42,* 516–526.

Vance, C. (1999). Mentoring: The nursing leader and mentor's perspective. In C. A. Sanerson (Ed.), *Nursing student to leader: The critical path to leadership development* (pp. 200–211). Albany, NY: Delmar.

Vance, C., & Olson, R. (Eds.). (1998). *The mentor connection in nursing.* New York: Springer Publishing.

Yoder, L. (1990). Mentoring: A concept analysis. *Nursing Administration Quarterly, 15,* 9–19.

Zachary, L. (2002). *The mentor's guide.* San Francisco: Jossey-Bass.

CHAPTER 3

Empowering Versus Enabling

One way leaders empower and assist others to empower themselves is by respecting each person and the person's ability to contribute to an organization and the profession. Certain variables such as the organizational culture, the leadership style of the nurse and other administrators, and the current collaborative practice or faculty governance model have an impact on how empowered nurses can be in their work setting. Due to the high patient acuity and demand for nurses and the scarce resources in both practice and academia, the environment is ripe for nurse leaders to think creatively about new ways to accomplish work. In this way, they can both use their leadership ability and help to empower others to capture what they want to do to make a difference in their everyday work, their career path, and for the nursing profession. It is necessary for nurses to increase their autonomy in the clinical arena, gain momentum in carving out areas of research that will strengthen nursing science, add to evidence-based practice, and network together to create partnerships to fulfill both clinical and academic missions. This chapter describes the concept of empowerment; strategies to help empower oneself, others, and the profession; a comparison of empowerment with the enabling process; and how creating a mentoring culture will empower the profession.

EMPOWERMENT

Empowerment means being inspired with self-confidence and the knowledge that one can make a difference by one's actions. It eventually leads to increased self-esteem. *Empowering*, or being able to empower others, is defined as being able to encourage an individual or oneself with confidence and demonstrating the ability to pass a sense of authority to another person or oneself. It is exactly what nurses need rather than being enabled to fulfill orders from members of other disciplines. The hierarchical structure that has existed for decades is changing, and staff nurses, advanced practice nurses, and nurse administrators are assuming more equitable positions of authority. Wheatley (1999), in explaining the new science of leadership, recommends empowering all and decreasing the constraints of bureaucratic structures in order to improve productivity and quality. This paradigm change supports people in achieving higher self-esteem as an outcome of feeling more self-confident in their work setting.

To improve understanding, one should be able to differentiate between self-confidence and self-esteem. Self-confidence encompasses how an individual feels at a given time and can be affected by many variables, such as one's health or even the weather. Self-esteem is a constant feeling of acceptance for the person one is. It is not influenced by everyday events. It is a way of being.

Many (Glass, 1998; Glennon, 1992; Lee, 2000; Luna & Cullen, 1996) suggest that certain steps need to occur before an individual or group can become empowered. For example, imagine an orthopedic unit where the surgeons never communicate with the staff and continue to send them unstable postoperative patients and multiple admissions without bothering to develop any clinical protocols to follow. The surgeons and technicians treat the nurses with no respect and no recognition for their work. If the attitude were to change in a setting like this, nurses would have to be able to recognize the negative atmosphere they were working in and at the same time be aware that this type of demeaning environment was not present on most other nursing units. So the staff would need to be conscious of its poor work setting. Second, the nurses would need to be extremely competent with their knowledge and expertise in their clinical specialty, as well as have effective communication skills so they would have strong self-esteem. Finally, the staff would have to be resourceful enough to be able to negotiate with the administration and persuade them to listen and allow the nurses to confront the physicians in order to create a new work atmosphere.

Empowerment of an organization's workers is considered one of the most important aspects of whether an organization achieves excellence (Grossman & Valiga, 2005). All individuals need to feel successful and self-directed. Glennon (1992) has found that many nurses seem to reach for perfection that is basically unattainable in most health care delivery systems today. Nurses need to be recognized for the small wins that staff members achieve every day. This would serve to encourage the profession and give nurses hope that things can change. The unit or department also needs to get away from the idea that perfection is the goal or that nothing is ever good enough. So instead of always accentuating the negative, it is wise to focus on a more positive overall stance. Perhaps then staff will begin to think, act, and behave like winners.

Nurses need to be empowered themselves so that they can help their patients by empowering them to feel they can speak up about their condition and plan of care. Kodish et al. (2004) have found that when researchers talk with families in clinical trials who have children with leukemia, it helps to have a nurse on hand to reinforce the information and explain and answer questions. These researchers believe that having a nurse available "may reflect the benefits of better emotional support for parents at a difficult time allowing for parents to feel empowered enough to speak up, ask questions, and seek clarification" about their child. Empowering patients and their families is a high-level leadership skill that nurses who are self-empowered can do successfully.

Surely times have changed, and nurses today portray a much different image than when "nurses felt rooted in a calling of devotional service and self-sacrificial love, now seen as either repressed middle class women with psychological complexes or women held down as handmaidens of the patriarchal medical establishment" (Bradshaw, p. 472, 1995). Fortunately, empowered nursing leaders have emerged and transformed the profession to seek evidence-based knowledge that is now driving clinical practice, education, and nursing research. This new nursing practice defies the historical roots of the profession's actions and propels nursing toward a better future (Roberts & Vasquez, 2004).

Hillary Clinton (2002), along with Senator Gordon Smith, introduced the Nurse Reinvestment Act, which gives some long-overdue respect for nursing by offering seed money to hospitals to implement practices that recognize and maximize the value of nursing. This recognition involves having nurses contribute to decisions affecting policy and patient care and supporting nurses' continuing education and career advancement. Kouzes and Posner (1995) describe five sets of behavioral practices that have assisted leaders to become empowered and able to encourage people to do extraordinary things:

- Demonstrate perseverance.
- Have a focus or direction.
- Empower others.
- Be a role model.
- Recognize others' contributions.

Leadership is a skill that can be developed by coaching and through experiential learning. Kouzes and Posner remind us that leadership is everyone's business, and therefore everyone should accept the leadership challenge on a daily basis.

Meleis (2003) wrote in her editorial in the *Journal of Nursing Scholarship* that there are multiple ways to define empowerment. One example she shares is what the United States and other developed countries are doing when they recruit nurses from less developed countries to work as nurses. It is a form of empowerment for these nurses to have the choice of where they would like to work. Her perspective of empowerment involves giving nurses opportunities to use high technology, work in best-practice environments, increase their earning power, expand their education and knowledge base, and improve their family's situation. Certainly these nurses are able to enjoy improved working conditions and improve their own economic earning power. This perspective can be a win-win situation for all by empowering the foreign nurses and their families, as well as the health care system in the developed country.

STRATEGIES TO EMPOWER ONESELF AND OTHERS

Another way to view empowerment is as "an interpersonal process of providing the resources, tools, and environment to develop, build, and increase ability and effectiveness of others to set and reach goals for individual and social ends" (Hokanson-Hawks, 1992, p. 610). A significant point is the fact that nurses who do not have the resources to perform their job, no matter how good their self-esteem is and how aware they are of their poor situation, will not be able to complete their work. This aspect of empowerment, however, is generally assumed—that is, that nurses will have the basic resources to perform their work. Also significant for nurse empowerment is the idea that employers are often challenged to motivate their employees. So how do managers increase employee motivation and effectiveness? This question is always challenging to managers. What is the best method to use to increase work performance in others? How does one motivate someone else? These are tough questions that have always concerned managers.

Jon Katzenbach (2003) writes extensively on employee motivation and how to best tap unused employee capabilities by empowering them. Energizing people to do their best work so as to accomplish higher goals than anyone thought possible is what happens when the group is empowered.

Katzenbach presents five paths for energizing a workforce to generate high performance. He advocates that before choosing one of the paths, leaders conduct three reviews:

1. Review each of the five paths that can lead to having an emotionally committed, high-performing workforce. Identify what each has in common. Describe their differences. Brainstorm what conditions would favor following one path over another.
2. Determine why so many top-performing companies and institutions (the author presents in his book findings from studying several companies such as Southwest Airlines, Marriott, and Microsoft) follow different paths. Describe how the company was successful.
3. Determine how companies decide which path to follow.

These are Katzenbach's five paths:

1. Mission, Values, and Pride. This path is favored by companies that have successful teams with a history of employee pride. There must be value-driven leadership. Some groups that align with this path are the U.S. Marine Corps and Marriott International.
2. Process and Metrics. This path best serves companies with maturing marketplace conditions that pride themselves for having continuous improvement. They are driven by a dynamic market and large customer base. Examples of groups using this path are Avon Manufacturing, Hill's Pet Nutrition, and Johnson Controls.
3. Entrepreneurial Spirit. These groups thrive on high-risk, high-reward opportunities. There are significant employee ownership possibilities. The groups are rapidly growing and enjoy a dynamic market. Most have magnetic leaders with ambitious visions for the companies. An example is Vail Ski School.
4. Individual Achievement. There are highly ambitious individuals employed in these groups, and individual achievement is of primary importance to the group. They tend to have an extremely dynamic marketplace and a huge customer base. Home Depot and First USA are examples of companies choosing this path.
5. Recognition and Celebration. It is critical that the average worker contributes. The labor pool tends to be unskilled with low monetary reward. The work itself tends not to be stimulating; however, there are magnetic leaders who trigger the energy of the workforce. Examples are Kentucky Fried Chicken and Southwest Airlines.

Katzenbach recommends that no matter what path is chosen, those in administration have to demonstrate that "they really care about each worker, and they have to honestly believe that he or she matters to the performance of the enterprise" (p. 236). He also notes that although each organization that he studied focused predominantly on one path, they tended to use other paths as supplements to accomplishing work goals. It is imperative to realize that in order to empower employees to be top performers, the leader-administrator must know how to generate emotional energy, how to channel the energy to be effective, and instill the discipline needed to maintain energy and commitment at such extraordinary levels. This model for motivating employees is very conducive for mentoring.

In *Why Pride Matters More Than Money*, Katzenbach (2003) dangles the infamous carrot on the front cover of his book. He believes emotional commitment from employees is the key to success and keeping competitive. Pride in one's work and recognition are significant rewards that nurses are seeking today. Many think that monetary reward is what it takes to motivate employees, but this is only part of it. Katzenbach (2003) repeatedly talks about pride. He feels that in order to be successful and perform at a high level, one needs a strong ego as well as self-serving pride. Nursing, in any specialty area, is a high-performance job. If nurses can (1) feel proud of themselves and (2) have those they respect and admire feel proud of them, two motivational dimensions are satisfied. Katzenbach challenges all "leaders in almost any organizational setting to motivate higher employee performance by capitalizing on the anticipation of feeling proud and making others proud, too" (p. 3). He believes that development of pride-building skills can be learned and can build long-term sustainability for an organization. In addition, cultivating pride in the nursing workforce can propel the nursing profession to bigger and better things.

Risher (2003) lists four "common sense" ways of improving employee performance: (1) get the employees to work harder; (2) train them with better work methods to be more productive; (3) try to reengineer the way the work is done, and then train them again; and (4) empower the workers to develop better methods. Empowering employees involves trust, and once there is trust between the management and the employees, there will be increased performance. This is a new empowerment philosophy that recognizes what employees have to offer more so than ever before. Also the idea of Total Quality Management, introduced by Deming (1994), assisted in demonstrating that frontline workers play a major role in solving quality problems. Alongside this new paradigm of thinking regarding the trusting of the worker came a new focus on employee commitment, which Becker, Ulrich, and Houselid (2001) describe as "engagement plus dedication," meaning that employees who are committed to the goals of the organization and have pride in their work will be intentionally engaged and willing to put in discretionary energy to accomplish their work goals. It is important to have employees who are committed to the organization and the profession and not just to their own careers. Nurses, both mentors and mentees, can role model-empowering behavior by

- being positive and proactive;
- giving control to frontline employees;
- offering culturally sensitive assistance;
- encouraging individuals and recognizing all of the person's existing strengths;
- increasing awareness of available support systems;
- attempting to convey a joint sense of responsibility for work so a person does not become stressed;
- promoting the use of coping strategies to prevent a sense of panic;
- helping the person not only see that problems have been solved or needs met but that the person functioned as an active, responsible agent who played a significant role (Dunst & Trivette, 1987).

Books such as *101 Careers in Nursing* (Novotny, Lippman, Sanders, & Fitzpatrick, 2004) are resources to assist nurses and student nurses to make changes in their life through empowerment. Sullivan (2003) writes that becoming influential can be learned. In her book, *How to Be Influential as a Nurse*, she discusses strategies and the rules of the game to assist nurses in enhancing their skills so they can become more influential wherever they work and in whatever position they hold. Becoming more influential is empowering. Hudacek's *A Daybook for Nurses: Making a Difference Each Day* (2004) explains how nurses have been empowered by their patients or the patients' families to make a difference that not only assisted one patient but made a difference for many patients. An excellent example that clearly depicts someone making a difference describes a nurse who put an unstable premature twin in the newborn nursery bassinet with her stable, healthier twin to comfort and support her. The outcome was positive, and today this practice is universally implemented in neonatal intensive care units throughout the country.

Houser and Player (2004) recount the careers of 12 nurses (including Luther Christman, Gretta Styles, Loretta Ford, and Sue Donalson) who became leaders in the profession. Miller (2003) presents ideas on developing a résumé to best portray one's expertise, skill set, and experiences. Miller (2002) also feels that just writing down one's abilities assists in improving one's self-confidence. He suggests that nurses practice their interviewing skills with each other or an adviser prior to seeking a position. He advocates that students receive mentoring in three areas:

1. Developmental (self-esteem, social skills, motivation, attitude, and behavioral changes)
2. Work related (individual goals, work skills) and subject (lifelong learning philosophy, career)
3. General academic goals

Sirgo and Coeling (2005) suggest that new graduates should assess the work culture of organizations they are interested in working for. They point to the importance of evaluating organizational culture and describe this as "how things are done around here." They suggest using their tool as a framework in evaluating the work environment.

There are innovative ways to manage a career, such as having multiple career paths instead of just one job, working per diem to gain skills in a new clinical area, getting involved with health teaching outside the health care structure such as teaching first aid at a marina, offering cardiopulmonary resuscitation certification for police or interested civilians, managing a Web site that answers new mothers' questions on infant care, writing a column in a newspaper or magazine, participating in research trial evaluations, or learning sales techniques to market pharmaceuticals or high-technology equipment.

Gilley and Boughton (1996) describe how the manager yields control to the staff and how this empowers both staff and the manager. "Self-esteeming" is a two-way process between two individuals. Increased self-confidence occurs after receiving positive evaluations from one's supervisor or colleagues. This, in turn, increases one's self-esteem. This self-esteeming for the employee takes the relationship to a much deeper level: "In return for receiving some control, the employee must now challenge and stimulate the manager with regard to his or her role and responsibility, which will create a higher level of confidence for the manager" (p. 85–86). This is termed *reciprocal self-esteem*. It is an example of how nurses and managers can be synergistic and accomplish more at the same time that they improve staff morale. These authors offer a tool for measuring nurses' self-esteem as well as a checklist to determine outcomes of mentor-mentee relationships.

It is significant that the mentor or leader/manager also is empowered through the self-esteeming process. This process does not work if the nurse manager or mentor thinks, "I am only a nurse." Or, "My nurses need to follow the doctor's orders period." Or, "There is no need to call and ask about that patient; just follow the protocol that Dr. Lisa gave us." In fact, someone who is not empowered has no possibility of empowering, let alone assisting others to empower themselves. Shaffer, Tallarico, and Walsh (2000, p. 36) remind us that mentoring can assist colleagues who may feel "powerless and insignificant" in their health care system to gain pride and self-confidence from their mentoring and from the mentee. If there is a network of multiple mentors, along with peer mentoring, the culture of mentoring can become pervasive. Mentors gain leadership and teaching skills and rekindle their pride in the profession through a novice's eyes. Also institutions are more likely to retain nurses who are feeling valued and empowered. However, Burke, Boal, and Mitchell (2004), Espelan and Shanta (2001), and Luna and Cullen (1996), among others, feel a mentor must want to be a mentor in order to be successful and feel they are part of the empowerment process of new employees and peers. It stands to reason that individuals who are not willing to mentor or who are manipulative will work against developing a mentoring culture in a unit.

Yeomans (1990) echoes what we all know to be true: the more one orders a person to do something a certain way, the better the chance is that it will be done in a less acceptable way. It is obvious that using a participatory leadership style, not an autocratic, one will best create an environment conducive to empowering the staff. As Blanchard and Johnson (1982) describe in their classic work, *The One Minute Manager*, people who feel good about who they are produce the best results.

Worrell, McGinn, Black, Holloway, and Ney (1996) propose the following model for faculty to role-model in order to provide empowerment to students, who will thereby become collegial, effective communicators, autonomous, and accountable:

Collegiality.   The relationship should be based on mutual respect for all involved. Faculty need to give honest feedback to students and not offer false praise in order to please them. Faculty should coach the students in order to use all of their potential. This acts to empower them. Faculty can also mentor their students by role-modeling political survival skills (Glass, 1998).

Communication.   Faculty need to effectively transmit information to all involved. There must be opportunities for students to engage in dialogue with their professors. Faculty cannot just provide all of the information that students need to learn. There must be interactive learning. Students who are spoon-fed information will be enabled and will not develop self-confidence.

Autonomy.   Students need to be independent. They need to learn problem-solving skills so they can think critically and have supervised practice in providing solutions to problems they encounter. Having autonomy will also increase student self-esteem.

Accountability.   Students must be responsible for their actions as well as their learning. Faculty or supervisor must not allow students to be rescued. They need to be held accountable for their actions. Faculty and supervisors who are codependent will offer unsolicited advice or enable a student who is actually capable of handling his or her own challenges.

Table 3.1 presents some suggestions for individuals to use in order to increase their leadership skills and become or remain empowered.

Glennon (1992) suggests using a model that allows for maximum nurse empowerment and participation. Optimism, respect, trust, and mutual goal formation are the foundational components. It is comparable to prototypes in *The One Minute Manager* by Blanchard and Johnson (1982). Success with this model revolves around developing an atmosphere of respect and recognition for the nurse. DiMeglio et al. (2005) describe a mentor program they are developing that concentrates on socializing new nurses. They discuss solutions regarding some of the issues that new nurses face, such as negative communication, generational differences, accountability, and peer competence.

Empowerment is exactly what nurses need rather than being enabled to fulfill what the physician and others order for patients. The hierarchical

TABLE 3.1   Practice Strategies to Increase Staff Empowerment

- Before registering a complaint, try to configure a possible solution that can be submitted along with the complaint.
- Stop whining about everything new. Be flexible, or at least try the change.
- Assess the pros and cons of the situation, and attempt to outweigh the cons.
- Prioritize one's battles. Focus on only the two most important ones.
- Review your colleagues' strengths.
- Review your own strengths.
- Avoid the doom and gloom. Try smiling, which releases endorphins and improves your overall well-being.
- Set a positive tone, and try to avoid peer pressure (when everyone agrees to something because someone else does and now are too tired to reflect comprehensively on the issue).
- Network, and keep abreast of grassroot opinions.

structure that has existed for decades is changing, and staff nurses, advanced practice nurses, and nurse administrators are assuming more equitable positions of authority. Wheatley (1999) explains the new science of leadership and recommends empowering all and decreasing the constraints of bureaucratic structures. This organizational movement will generate higher-quality outcomes and improved patient care, and therefore increasing productivity and decreasing costs, while improving the work environment. Among the benefits generated when there is nurse empowerment are improved patient care, increased nurse professionalism, and expanded nurse problem-solving ability (Espeland & Shanta, 2001).

ENABLING

Enabling is a perpetuation of the status quo and maintaining nurse dependency. Behavior that prevents an individual from acquiring new competencies, decreases one's sense of control over life, and reinforces old, maladaptive behaviors such as passivity and procrastination reflect enabling (Dunst & Trivette, 1987). In fact, enabling is defined by the field of drug and alcohol addiction as allowing or encouraging the drug dependence to continue or even worsen. Essentially enabling is part of codependency. Someone who is codependent manifests behaviors of assuming others' responsibility, taking care of others' needs, and rescuing others from the consequences of their behaviors. Faculty, managers, and colleagues can be guilty of protecting and rescuing certain students and nurses. Enabling is clearly described as "behaviors by others that perpetuates dependent behaviors" (Haber, Krainovich-Miller, McMahon, & Price-Hoskins, 1997, p. 516).

Enabling leads to people feeling entitled, that is, believing they should receive an honor or recognition because of the work they put into a project, or in preparing for a specific role in a play, or in practicing for selection to an elite athletic competition. One may hear nurses say, "I have paid my dues and refuse to work another Christmas holiday; let the new people do the holidays." This is a projection of feeling entitled and may be a result of having been enabled. Rather, leaders need to empower students and nurses by teaching them to handle their own responsibilities, assisting them to become independent, and maintaining the policies of the hospital or health care agency or school of nursing so they have to face the consequences of their actions. Faculty must provide opportunities for students to do their own problem solving and be accountable for them; otherwise, student self-esteem will suffer, and they will never become empowered.

RECOGNITION AND PRIDE

Kouzes and Posner (2003) suggest that people who are recognized for their good work and are encouraged are more likely to achieve higher levels of success. They recommend strategies for leaders to use to support others' need to be appreciated for what they do. They explain "encouraging the heart" as consisting of four components:

- Leaders must follow general principles that reward employees for work well done.
- Leaders will not be perceived as being soft for encouraging the heart. In fact, in order to fulfill stretch goals, it is essential to follow the heart.
- Various leaders have multiple methods they use to encourage the heart.
- All leaders must be aware of the soul and spirit involved in any organization.

Just as Sinetar (1998) describes mentoring as the art of encouragement and soul, Kouzes and Posner (2003) note that an extremely important component of empowering staff is to "encourage the heart," such as the encouragement a mentor gives. This encouragement of the heart is often what is missing in the work environment of nurses yet is a spirit that fits with advancing a mentoring culture in nursing.

Mentors and preceptors can assist their colleagues in gaining leadership skills by giving them opportunities to practice effective communication, administrative tasks, team building, conflict management, and supervision of other employees—for example, by

- taking positions that offer new and increased responsibilities;
- managing special start-up assignments that afford them visibility;
- handling personnel problems like conflicts and firings;
- representing the unit at a division or departmental meeting;
- leading a unit staff meeting;
- scheduling and managing staff work requests for the next three-month period;
- developing an interdisciplinary clinical protocol;
- meeting with members of outside health care agencies to set up a partnership.

Goode et al. (1993) studied (N = 322) staff nurses' perception of job satisfaction and found 92% identified recognition as the most significant reason for feeling satisfied with position. Twenty-eight percent felt recognition was seldom or never given. In another study ($N = 239$), hospital nurses identified the most meaningful recognition as verbal feedback, most commonly given by nurse manager. Four main reasons prompted staff nurse recognition: outstanding performance or patient care delivery; expertise, assuming additional responsibilities, or involvement in professional activities; receiving a certification or degree; and years of service. Other ways of receiving recognition include the opportunity to serve on a task force, receiving additional training to share with peers, preceptorship, participation in unit orientation, involvement in planning for patient care or the unit operation, having charge nurse responsibilities, or an invitation to speak at a professional meeting. Blegan et al. (1992) studied nurses' perceptions of the most meaningful recognition ($N = 341$). Findings included monetary rewards commensurate with performance, private verbal feedback, and written acknowledgment by the nurse manager

MENTORING CULTURE

Bernhard and Walsh (1990) provide an interesting four-stage model that integrates and substantiates the close relationship between mentoring, empowerment, and motivating individuals:

Stage 1, Input: Employees must have inner motivation in order for mentoring and empowerment to occur.

Stage 2, Process: Through mentoring, energy can be channeled to accomplish goals and increase mentees' perceptions of the environment. Both the mentor and mentee become motivated to achieve their own goals.

Stage 3, Output: The goal of mentoring is for the mentee to become empowered. This prepares the mentee to be accountable.

Stage 4, Feedback: The empowered mentee will acquire high self-esteem and competence. It is time for the mentee to mentor and attempt to motivate someone else.

This model could be helpful for managers to use when illustrating the process a mentor and mentee can expect with the progression of a mentoring relationship. It also spells out the cyclic nature of mentoring on a unit or department. The stages of input, process, output, and feedback can be put on a horizontal continuum and dated so that the mentor and mentee have target dates for their completion of the mentorship.

It is imperative that nurses be empowered to become leaders, and mentoring can strengthen this initiative. Lee (2000) relates that until recently, power was most frequently perceived as something to acquire and generally at the expense of another who may have had the power. This is no longer true. Rather, a new perception of power transfer has emerged: that power can be shared to help others. This is the essence of empowerment. In order to empower nurses on a unit, a nurse manager has to provide mentoring relationships and give nurses freedom to use their creativity to generate new ideas and accomplish goals. "Empowered nurses become role models for others and enrich themselves through coaching and sharing power" (p. 26). Lee supports the idea that mentoring, empowerment, and motivation are all part of a synergistic relationship. Studies conducted by Aiken, Clarke, Sloane, Sochalski, and Siber (2002) and Needleman, Buerhaus, Mattke, Stewart, and Zelevinsky (2002) document that nurses need to be more collaborative with peers and other members of the health care team, more autonomous with their decision making, and more capable of providing strong leadership. How better to learn collaboration skills, gain self-confidence, increase decision-making ability, and develop leadership than to work with a coach or mentor?

Shaffer, Tallarico, and Walsh (2000) suggest the following actions be included in order for successful empowerment of mentor and mentee during the traditional stages of the mentoring relationship:

1. Initiation.   During this initial time, the two people should determine the other's qualities that interest each in forming the mentorship. For example, what strengths and networks does the mentor have? What potential does the mentor see in the mentee? What is in it for the mentor? Ideas for establishing goals are discussed.

2. Cultivation.   The relationship is defined with specific goals and activities that will benefit both mentor and mentee. Are there any connections that the mentor or mentee may have to expedite the accomplishments of goals? Schedules are made that are mutually agreed on by both the mentor and mentee.

3. Separation.   Some mentorships end spontaneously, but most that are successful enter this phase, and both the mentor and the mentee gradually dissolve or limit the relationship. Often one of the two experiences a career move that separates them geographically, but they remain in a long-term relationship in spite of the distance. They continue to assist each other with career advancement and are now more like colleagues, both being equally empowered.

4. Redefinition.   This stage varies with each pair, and some relationships never proceed to this stage because they just ended. It is difficult to know if the mentee or mentor were ever empowered if the mentoring relationship did not progress and faded away. Others become colleagues and enjoy success from their relationship. There is little advice being given at this point since the pair have most likely become peers who are equally empowered and are both richer for their mentorship.

One program for senior nurse executives, the Executive Nurse Fellows Program, for the Robert Wood Johnson Foundation developed by the Center for the Health Professions at the University of California, San Francisco, has been experimenting with the most effective ways nurses can change their skill set in order to more fully participate in delivering health care. Nurses need to be prepared to assist with the reintegration of psychosocial behavioral aspects of care with the traditional biomedical ones, design of creative teams to participate effectively in care delivery systems, and redesign of care delivery systems to maximize patient outcomes.

The Leadership Program described by O'Neil and Morjikian (2003) encompasses five competencies that each executive (and nurses wishing to increase their leadership skills) must master during the fellowship:

1. *Self-knowledge*, defined as the ability to develop the self in the context of organizational challenges and interpersonal demands.
2. *Interpersonal communication effectiveness*, which encompasses the ability to translate a vision and motivate followers. Followers engage in exercises to assist them in understanding how they are perceived by others.
3. *Risk taking and creativity*, so as to move beyond what has worked in the past and develop transformational changes to move the organization to success.
4. *Inspiring change* in order to steer the organization in an entirely different way that provides maximum effectiveness.
5. *Strategic vision for the future*, so that connections between social, economic, and political issues are a part of the organization's long-term plan.

Participants use self-ratings and peer and supervisor ratings to gather data to map out a development plan for their year as a fellow. Coaches as well as other fellows and peers assist each other in determining their plan of leadership development. Lombardo and Eichinger (1996) give some specific strategies for the fellow as well as the coaches and mentors in their book, *For Your Improvement: A Development and Coaching Guide*. Although this is designed as an advanced leadership program for nurse executives in health services, public health, and nursing education, anyone can gain leadership skills by practicing these strategies, and mentors can role-model them for mentees.

Cox (1991) researched the perception of staff and managers' idea of leadership evident in a health care agency and found that nurses perceived an autocratic style in which managers saw a participatory style of leadership. What nurse managers may feel they are exemplifying is not always perceived similarly by staff. This is a good reason to participate in a leadership development seminar in order to attain feedback on how one's communication and leadership style are perceived by others. Certainly among the biggest challenges nurses face are communication and collaboration problems. Burke et al. (2004) cite two studies indicating that nurses and physicians have difficulty with communicating. Thomas, Sexton, and Helmreich (2003) found a "difference between nurse and physician perceptions of communication among health care members. They found that 73% of the physicians felt there was high quality of collaboration with nurses, but only 33% of the nurses agreed that they had high-quality collaboration with physicians. Rosenstein (2002) found with 1200 responses from employees of 84 hospitals or medical groups in the Veterans Hospital Agency West Coast network that there was a discrepancy between nurses and physicians regarding the professional atmosphere at their facilities. There was a statistically significant difference, with physicians feeling they enjoyed good collaboration and nurses feeling they did not. In fact, 30% of respondents felt they knew at least one nurse who had left the institution because of disruptive, noncollegial physician behavior.

Other leadership programs, such as the American Colleges of Collegiate Nursing and the Helene Fuld Foundation, sponsor a year-long leadership fellowship for nurse faculty interested in becoming deans and directors of nursing programs. Approximately 50 fellows are selected annually and attend two 3-day workshops in Washington, D.C., where they participate in leadership development groups and work with a dean mentor throughout the year (for information on the fellowship and application process, go to www.aacn.nche.edu). This fellowship affords the opportunity for leadership assessment and evaluation, networking, and consultation with mentor to achieve long-term goals.

International mentoring through the Chiron Mentor-Fellow Program is another mentoring program that will advance nursing as well as individual nurses. Sigma Theta Tau International (STTI) offers members the opportunity to work with mentors and develop leadership skills in a formalized fellowship through the Chiron Mentor-Fellow Program. During a 12-month program, nurses who desire skill development in specific leadership areas are guided by experienced mentors as they implement individualized plans and participate in group activities. Potential mentors and fellows are encouraged to seek out partners and apply as a pair to the Chiron Mentor-Fellow program. (For applications, go to www.nursingsociety .org or e-mail leadership@stti.iupui.edu.) STTI sponsors the Chiron Leadership Mentoring Program that provides leadership development opportunities for nurses.

Aiken et al. (2002) and Needleman et al. (2002) document that nurses need to be more collaborative with peers and other members of the health care team, more autonomous with their decision making, and more capable of providing strong leadership. Mentors can assist leaders to become empowered and be more collaborative, autonomous, and better leaders. Mentorships assist nurses in gaining insight into their ability to lead change, think creatively, empower themselves as well as others, and acquire skills to prepare them for a successful career and strengthen the nursing profession. Nurses identify that it is most significant for the nurse manager and other leaders to portray caring in order to have an environment conducive to staff empowerment (Peterson, 1990). Koloroutis (2004) agrees that caring is a significant attribute of an effective leader and describes how work settings can be more caring focused in her book, *Relationship Based Care: A Model for Transforming Practice*. Risher (2003) points out that the biggest problem for managers is to have employees who do not care about the success of the organization. This disengagement can be identified easily by looking for the people who put in their time and go home. Approximately one out of three employees feel this way. No one wants them as employees, but they can be found in every workplace (Risher, 2003).

Mentoring should be institutionalized as an integral part of nursing practice—as a useful, honorable way of life of a fully functional professional nurse (Werner, 2002). Having a mentor can greatly assist every nurse to develop leadership ability. Nurses need to have good relationships among themselves in order to be a successful team. Team building must be focused on performance results and not just becoming a team. Katzenbach and Smith (1999) present basic rules for team building in their best-seller, *The Wisdom of Teams: Creating the High-Performance Organization*:

1. Have no more than 12 people on any team to ensure effectiveness.
2. The team must have a common purpose.
3. There must be a common set of specific performance goals.

4. There must be a commonly agreed-on working approach.
5. All members must hold one another mutually accountable for their performance.

The authors say that teams outperform individuals especially when performance requires multiple talents and experience. And although most people agree that teams almost always outperform individuals, they generally overlook opportunities to participate in teams, especially those in higher-level positions. The authors quote Jack Welch, former chief executive officer of General Electric, who says: "Change is in the air. General Electric people today understand the pace of change, the need for speed, the absolute necessity of moving more quickly in everything we do. . . . Every effort of every man and woman in the company is focused on satisfying customers' needs. Internal functions begin to blur. Customer service? It's not somebody's job. It's everybody's job" (p. 17).

Nurses need to get back to serving the customer. We all can benefit from working in teams, and Katzenbach and Smith (1999) explain why teams perform so well. First, working in a team brings together skills, experience, and knowledge that surpass what any one individual has. Second, a team can accomplish goals more quickly than any one individual. Third, teams are cost-effective. And finally, teams bring socialization into the work setting and tend to provide opportunities for fun, which solidifies the team further. Teams are related to networks, and as we know, networking triggers success in most people's work settings as well as careers. Coaches and mentors, such as clinical nurse specialists, staff development directors, and other department and special project directors, have a key role in assisting these teams to produce the maximum performance possible.

Stone (1999) offers some critical skills for team coaching:

- *Defining.* Direct the team to identify purpose and goals.
- *Summarizing.* Summarize the team's progress at each milestone, and bring the team together to rework goals and evaluate work as necessary.
- *Facilitating.* Keep the team spirit alive by encouraging dialogue, but be sure not to assume leadership of the team. Stay in the facilitator role.
- *Organizing.* Distribute agendas, plan meetings, circulate minutes, and keep the team on track for accomplishing its goals.
- *Developing.* Role-model the skills the team needs in order to work together to accomplish its goals.

How better to accomplish this than by role-modeling for the new nurses, allowing nurses to shadow each other, providing a strong precepting program for skill orientation, and having a manager and staff who recognize each other's strengths and competencies? As Wheatley says, "What gives power its charge, positive or negative, is the quality of the relationships" (1999, p. 40). Nurses need to role-model more for each other the positive ways of communicating and managing conflict so that all nurses can be empowered to stand up and say what is really bothering them or what they would like to see happen where they work. This positive role modeling can generate an atmosphere in which nurses want to be mentored and choose to mentor. Growth will be encouraged and nurtured, and self-empowerment of nurses will be visible. This increased leadership ability of all nurses will increase patient care quality, cost-effectiveness, and nurse retention. Ultimately, the power demonstrated by each individual will be multiplied as more and more networking generates collaboration, which will undoubtedly produce a more influential overall effect (Gilbert, 1995)

So too, empowerment of a mentee is crucial to the success of a mentorship. However, the mentor must be self-empowered as evidenced by exhibiting self-esteem and a positive self-image, being a risk taker and not dependent on the approval of others, having positive expectations, and being able to interact with others effectively (Lloyd & Berthelot, 1992). Many truly empowered and effective leaders say, "I have completed my job here when you no longer need me," which means the employees have become empowered.

CONCLUSION

Empowerment is necessary for all nurses as well as for the advancement of the profession of nursing. As leaders develop, they become more self-empowered and able to empower others. Nurses must gain self-confidence, a goal that can be achieved by becoming competent with both clinical skills and leadership skills such as negotiation, creative thinking, communication, and collaboration. In order to achieve this confidence, nurses need to be mentored by experienced nurses who can provide knowledge, psychosocial support, and networking. Mentors can assist individuals to increase their self-confidence, and in time, their self-esteem will heighten. By affording opportunities for nurses to empower themselves, practice leadership, and work with role models, coaches, and mentors, nurses will continue to make a difference in patient care.

REFERENCES

Aiken, L., Clarke, S., Sloane, D., Sochalski, J., & Siber, J. (2002). Hospital staffing and patient mortality, nurse burnout, and job dissatisfaction. *Journal of the American Medical Association, 288*, 1987–1993.

Becker, B., Ulrich, D., & Houselid, M. (2001). *The human resource scorecard: Linking people, strategy, and performance.* Boston: Harvard Business School Press.

Bernhard, L., & Walsh, M. (1990). *Leadership: The key to the professionalization of nursing* (2nd ed.). St. Louis: Mosby.

Blanchard, K., & Johnson, S. (1982). *The one minute manager.* New York: Berkeley.

Blegan, M., Goode, C., Johnson, M., Maas, M., McCloskey, J., & Moorhead, S. (1992). Recognizing staff nurse job performance and achievements. *Research in Nursing and Health, 15*, 57–66.

Bradshaw, A. (1995). What are nurses doing to patients? A review of theories of nursing past and present. *Journal of Clinical Nursing, 4*, 81–92.

Brennan, P. (2003). Mentoring and the Mentor Match Program. *Nursing in Focus, 4*, 6.

Burke, M., Boal, J., & Mitchell, R. (2004). Communicating for better care: Improving nurse-physician communication. *American Journal of Nursing, 104*, 40–47.

Byrne, M. (2003). A mentored experience (K01) in maternal-infant research. *Journal of Professional Nursing, 19*, 66–75.

Clinton, H. (2002). Respect: The not-so-secret ingredient. *American Journal of Nursing, 102*, 11.

Cox, H. (1991). Verbal abuse nationwide: part 1: Oppressed group behavior. *Nursing Management, 22*, 32–35.

Deming, W. E. (1994). *The new economics for industry, government, and education* (2nd ed.). Cambridge, MA: MIT Center for Advanced Engineering.

DiMeglio, K., Padula, C., Piatek, C., Korber, S., Barrett, A., Ducharme, M., et al. (2005). Group cohesion and nurse satisfaction: Examination of a team-building approach. *Journal of Nursing Administration, 35*, 110–120.

Dunst, C., & Trivette, C. (1987). Enabling and empowering families: Conceptual and intervention issues. *School Psychology Review, 16*, 443–456.

Espeland, K., & Shanta, L. (2001). Empowering versus enabling in academia. *Journal of Nursing Education, 40*, 342–346.

Gilbert, T. (1995). Nursing: Empowerment and the problem of power. *Journal of Advanced Nursing, 21*, 865–871.

Gilley, J., & Boughton, N. (1996). *Stop managing, start coaching.* Chicago: Irwin.

Glass, N. (1998). Becoming de-silenced and reclaiming voice: Women nurses speak out. In I. Kelleher & P. McInerney (Eds.), *Nursing matters* (pp. 127–137). Melbourne, Australia: Harcourt Brace.

Glennon, T. (1992). Empowering nurses through enlightened leadership. *Journal of Nurse Empowerment, 2*, 41–44.

Goode, C., Ibarra, V., Blegan, M., Anderson-Bruner, J., Boshart-Yoder, T., Cram, E., et al. (1993). What kind of recognition do staff nurses want? *American Journal of Nursing, 93*, 64–68.

Grossman, S., & Valiga, T. (2005). *The new leadership challenge: Creating the future of nursing* (2nd ed.). Philadelphia: F. A. Davis.

Haber, J., Krainovich-Miller, B., McMahon, A., & Price-Hoskins, P. (1997). *Comprehensive psychiatric nursing*. St. Louis: Mosby.

Hokanson-Hawks, J. (1992). Empowerment in nursing education: Concept analysis and application to philosophy, learning and instruction. *Journal of Advanced Nursing, 17,* 609–618.

Houser, B., & Player, K. (2004). *Pivotal moments in nursing: Leaders who changed the path of a profession*. Indianapolis, IN: STTI.

Hudacek, S. (2004). *A daybook for nurses: Making a difference each day*. Indianapolis, IN: Center Nursing Press.

Katzenbach, J. (2003). *Why pride matters more than money: The power of the world's greatest motivational force*. New York: Crown Business.

Katzenbach, J., & Smith, D. (1999). *The wisdom of teams: Creating the high performance organization* (2nd ed.). New York: HarperCollins.

Kodish, E., Eder, M., Noll, R. Ruccione, K., Lange, B., Angiolillo, A., et al. (2004). Communication of randomization in childhood leukemia trials. *Journal of American Medical Association, 291,* 470–475.

Koloroutis, K. (Ed.). (2004). *Relationship based care: A model for transforming practice*. Minneapolis: Creative Health Care Management.

Kouzes, J., & Posner, B. (1995). *The leadership challenge: How to keep getting extraordinary things done in organizations* (2nd ed.). San Francisco: Jossey-Bass.

Kouzes, J., & Posner, B. (2003). *Encouraging the heart: A leader's guide to rewarding and recognizing others* (2nd ed.). San Francisco: Jossey-Bass.

Lee, L. (2000). Motivation, mentoring, and empowerment aren't just management jargon—they're resources you use every day. *Nursing Management, 10,* 25–28.

Lloyd, S., & Berthelot, T. (1992). *Self empowerment*. Los Altos, CA: Crisp Publications.

Lombardo, M., & Eichinger, R. (1996). *For your improvement: A development and coaching guide*. Minneapolis: Lominger.

Luna, G., & Cullen, D. (1996). *Empowering the faculty: Mentoring redirected and renewed*. Washington, DC: George Washington University Press.

Meleis, A. (2003). Brain drain or empowerment? *Journal of Nursing Scholarship, 35,* 105.

Miller, A. (2002). *Mentoring students and young people*. Sterling, VA: Stylus Publishing.

Miller, T. (2003). *Building and managing a career in nursing: Strategies for advancing your career*. Indianapolis, IN: STTI.

Needleman, J., Buerhaus, P., Mattke, S., Stewart, M., & Zelevinsky, K. (2002). Nurse staffing levels and the quality of care in hospitals. *New England Journal of Medicine, 346,* 1715–1722.

Novotny, J., Lippman, D., Sanders, N., & Fitzpatrick, J. (2004). *101 careers in nursing*. New York: Springer Publishing.

O'Neil, E., & Morjikian, R. (2003). Nursing leadership: Challenges and opportunities. *Policy, Politics, and Nursing Practice, 4,* 173–179.

Peterson, K. (1990). Caring for people, not profits, brings success. *Modern Health Care, 20,* 34.

Risher, H. (2003). Tapping unused employee capabilities: How to create a high performance environment by changing the work paradigm. *Public Manager, 32,* 34–39.

Roberts, D., & Vasquez, E. (2004). Power: An application to the nursing image and advanced practice. *AACN Clinical Issues, 15,* 196–204.

Rosenstein, A. (2002). Original research: Nurse-physician relationships: Impact on nurse satisfaction and retention. *American Journal of Nursing, 102,* 26–34.

Shaffer, B., Tallarico, B., & Walsh, J. (2000). Win-win mentoring. *Dimensions of Critical Care Nursing, 6,* 36–38.

Sinetar, M. (1998). *The mentor's spirit: Life lessons on leadership and the art of encouragement.* New York: St. Martin's Press.

Sirgo, C., & Coeling, H. (2005). Work group culture and the new graduate. *American Journal of Nursing, 105,* 85–87.

Stone, F. (1999). *Coaching, counseling, and mentoring: How to choose and use the right technique to boost employee performance.* New York: AMACON.

Sullivan, E. (2003). *How to be influential as a nurse.* Upper Saddle River, NJ: Prentice Hall.

Thomas, E., Sexton, B., & Helmreich, R. (2003). Discrepant attitudes about teamwork among critical care nurses and physicians. *Critical Care Medicine, 31,* 956–959.

Werner, J. (2002). Mentoring and its potential nursing role. *Creative Nursing Journal, 3,* 13–14.

Wheatley, M. (1999). *Leadership and the new science: Discovering order in a chaotic world* (2nd ed.). San Francisco: Berrett-Koehler.

Worrell, J., McGinn, A., Black, E., Holloway, N., & Ney, P. (1996). The RN-BSN student: Developing a model of empowerment. *Journal of Nursing Education, 35,* 127–130.

Yeomans, W. (1990). *1000 things you never learned in business school.* New York: New American Library.

CHAPTER 4

Strategies for Developing Mentorships in Nursing

One Size Does Not Fit All

Mentoring is crucial and needs to be promoted among professional nurses and integrated into the nursing curriculum. It is important for individual nurses to identify skills they wish to work on and then choose someone to work with who possesses these attributes or skills. In order to prepare leaders, we must mentor them. Other leadership skills such as managing conflict, maintaining credibility, communicating effectively, taking risks, being flexible, being creative, having visions, and critically thinking are important for leaders to assist individuals in developing. Nurses will need to think about new ways of providing care. Collaboration, partnering, and networking skills will be important to acquire for these new health care delivery methods to be successful.

It is helpful to review the idea of a learning organization, which involves continuous dialogue between members of an institution. Senge, Kleiner, Roberts, Ross, and Smith remind us in their book, *The Fifth Discipline Fieldbook: Strategies and Tools for Building a Learning Organization*, that "a person is a person because of other people's acknowledgement" (1994, p. 3). Individuals who grow up with this idea that we all need others to successfully form our identity are aware of the need for creating a mentoring culture. Following are the five recommended learning disciplines for individuals to use to foster this team effort attitude:

1. Personal mastery: Encouraging members of organizational settings to develop themselves around their individual goals and purposes
2. Mental models: Attempting to continually clarify our internal picture of the world that influences our actions and decisions

3. Shared vision: Being part of a group by building a sense of commitment toward shared futures
4. Team learning: Honing thinking skills so that groups of people "can reliably develop intelligence and ability greater than the sum of individual members' talents" (p. 6)
5. Systems thinking: A way of rethinking about how forces and interrelationships shape the behavior of systems to be more synchronized with the larger processes of the world

Developing mentorships and preceptorships that reflect these five disciplines can be helpful in improving nurse morale and help to solidify the profession's contributions to health care. Leaders can make a difference by asking other nurses to follow a lifelong learning philosophy by modeling the behaviors in the five disciplines. In *Presence: Human Purpose and the Field of the Future* (2004), Senge, Scharmer, Jaworski, and Flowers share their ideas of collaboration and networking in order to create a preferred future. Nurses need direction in finding a way to create change and ultimately the future. One important belief is to acknowledge that nurses must work with others to be successful. Therefore, mentoring others through partnering initiatives will undoubtedly assist nurses to be more successful leaders and gain higher satisfaction with their lives. This chapter reviews characteristics for identifying successful mentors and mentees; describes effective mentoring and precepting models; differentiates mentorships, preceptorships, shadowing experiences, internships, and externships; presents ideas regarding best practice clinical preceptorships for graduate students; and offers ways to create culturally competent mentorships. However, since one size does not fit all, nurses need to be able to develop mentorships, preceptorships, and coaching styles to fit individuals and their situations. People vary according to their developmental stage, their level of competency, their leadership and followership styles, and in other ways. Even with preceptorships with prescribed orientation programs, the preceptor needs to individualize the program to the preceptee. This chapter discusses characteristics of effective mentors, mentees, and mentoring,

CHARACTERISTICS OF EFFECTIVE MENTORS AND MENTEES

To be successful with mentorships of any kind, it stands to reason that the individuals who are going to be the mentors or preceptors should be interested in mentoring or precepting others and possess certain character-istics. Tables 4.1 and 4.2, regarding mentoring with various models, are based on a review of the literature (Andrews & Wallis, 1999; Bennetts, 2000; Byrne & Keefe, 2003; Greene & Puetzer, 2002; Schwiebert, 2000; Snell, 1999; and Zachary, 2000). There is agreement that mentors who fit this classification can still be negative mentors if they are manipulative and in-compatible with their mentee. Some mentors may act as though everything is going along well with the mentoring but secretly abuse the mentee to ob-tain more mileage for their own career or even sabotage the mentee's career. Others may temporarily enable and protect a mentee who is not prepared sufficiently until enough time lapses that the mentor anticipates no positive outcomes coming from investing time and resources into the relationship. Some mentors view failure to mentor an individual successfully as their own failure and do not attribute it to the mentee or situation. Whether an inef-fective mentoring or precepting relationship will be identified by others or the organization depends on several variables. In the case of a preceptorship when the time involved is limited and the goal is focused on attaining skills for orientation to a particular position, it becomes more difficult to evaluate if a preceptor is really good. Another compounding variable with precepting is that preceptors generally have to precept new employees in order to main-tain their clinical ladder position or attain a promotion on the clinical lad-der. Having a mandate to precept can have a great impact on the relationship between the preceptor and preceptee since the preceptor in many instances has not voluntarily accepted this responsibility.

Luna and Cullen (1996) believe that not every individual is a good mentee and not every individual needs a mentoring relationship. Others (Bennetts, 2000; Schwiebert, 2000; Zachary, 2000) feel that everyone who has an effective mentor can benefit from this relationship. As previously discussed, most nurses have precepting relationships, not mentorships, and the precepting relationship has more of a skill-oriented focus over a defined period of time. Some preceptorships also focus on decision making and allow the preceptee to have continuous consultations with them even after the orientation period. So preceptees need to demonstrate satisfactory skills and decision-making ability in their preceptorship in order to complete their orientation to becoming a staff nurse. Due to the nature of a precep-torship, the preceptor and preceptee can generally work out any differ-ences, whereas the relationship between a mentor and mentee is more intricate, and the behavior and productivity of mentees have a more direct reflection on the mentor. It is most advantageous for the relationship if both parties possess the characteristics listed in Tables 4.1 and 4.2.

TABLE 4.1   Characteristics of Effective Mentors

Strong self-esteem and self-empowerment

Effective communication skills

Uninvested in preserving the status quo

Politically astute in the workplace environment

Able to balance personal and professional responsibilities

Respected in the workplace by peers and senior administrators

Highly knowledgeable in the field and interested in new challenges

Willing to volunteer to mentor someone and past experience with a good mentor

Previous effective mentoring experience

Mentor's workplace considers mentoring significant and valuable

Motivated to mentor well; there is incentive to be a good mentor, and resources provided for the mentor

TABLE 4.2   Characteristics of Effective Mentees

Comfortable and willing to participate in mentorship

Effective communication skills

Willing to receive constructive feedback and work under the direction of another

Goal driven and with goals that are compatible with the mentor's goals

An area of interest that is different from but compatible with the mentor's expertise

Determination to succeed and passionate about the profession

Responsible and able to be an independent decision maker when appropriate

Flexible and willing to participate in low-level work initially that may directly assist the mentor or organization and not necessarily the mentee

MENTORING, PRECEPTING, AND OTHER SUPPORT MODELS

There are no standard mentoring models used in nursing that are universally accepted (Smith, McAllister, & Crawford, 2001). Stages of mentoring have been described in Chapter 2 as including selection, goal setting, and working (Bower, 2000); recognition and development, limited independence, and termination and realignment (Fox & Shephard, 1998); and initiation, cultivation, separation, and redefinition (Kram, 1983). All seem to include similar components. Models in nursing do not correlate the stages of a mentoring relationship to the model. Rather, it is assumed that everyone proceeds through a model at their own pace or perhaps, in the case of preceptorships, over the period of time prescribed by the workplace for an orientation. Each setting needs to determine what works best for the purpose, time frame, and the resources set aside for the mentorship or preceptorship. The following six strategies suggested by Schwiebert (2000) are helpful to use for mentorship development:

1. Assess mentor strengths and networks, and determine how the mentee can fit into network and gain from the mentor's strengths. Mentors who have not been mentored may not be aware of the importance of using their network to assist the mentee. They also may be oblivious of their own strengths. It is often not the most famous professional who makes the most effective mentor.
2. Clarify expectations for the mentee and mentor. Both must articulate their expectations from the mentorship. Mentors should be sure not to base their goals for the mentee on their own achievements but on the mentee's potential.
3. Specific time needs to be scheduled for the mentor and mentee to meet regularly, and boundaries for the relationship need to be adhered to.
4. Support, encouragement, and constructive feedback need to be given to the mentee at regular intervals. Allow time for the mentee to respond to the feedback, and then assist the mentee in developing solutions.
5. Ensure that the mentee is invited to informal gatherings, and assist the individual in becoming part of a peer network or facilitate the individual to become part of a new network.
6. Review with the mentee the importance of participating fully in the relationship. Otherwise, the mentorship will not be successful in accomplishing the mentee's goals. The mentee must ensure he or she is doing what the mentor has recommended unless they have mutually agreed-on a change in the plan.

Typically mentees are looking for mentors who are direct with them, give positive and constructive feedback, are willing to share knowledge, are honest, are competent in their field, and are willing to let the mentee grow or become empowered. Preceptors can apply information from Schwiebert's (2000) six principles when developing an effective orientation program.

Zachary (2000) gives advice, worksheets, and exercises to assist in developing a mentoring program for any type of program and discipline. The following are his six suggestions:

1. Assess readiness to become a mentor.
2. Establish the mentor-mentee relationship.
3. Set appropriate goals.
4. Monitor progress and achievement.
5. Avoid common problems.
6. Conclude the mentoring relationship.

Zachary also provides fifteen ideas for program development design to assist in developing a program for one's organization:

1. Define the purpose.
2. Ensure viable support from top management.
3. Name the participants and the initiative.
4. Define the mentee pool.
5. Create the mentor pool.
6. Identify roles and responsibilities.
7. Develop the pairing protocol.
8. Build a mentor education and training program.
9. Identify ways to reward, recognize, and celebrate mentoring success.
10. Define management, oversight, and coordination.
11. Identify methods and procedures for tracking progress and providing for continuous improvement.
12. Plan the rollout or implementation.
13. Anticipate stumbling blocks and obstacles in the rollout process.
14. Plan the internal strategic communication campaign.
15. Anticipate mentoring casualties (affecting individual mentoring relationships).

Mentors, preceptors, and coaches need to be aware of cognitive learning styles, learning domains, and cultural competency. Benner's Skill Acquisition Model (1984) is a useful conceptual framework for developing mentorship models since it is used for clinical ladder programs. Some precepting programs are developed around Benner's model, which describes five stages that nurses experience as they develop through their careers:

1. Novice
2. Advanced beginner

3. Competent
4. Proficient
5. Expert

Generally, preceptors are in the competent through expert stages. Students are considered novices, and new graduates are advanced beginners. Due to the nursing shortage, there are not enough experts or proficient nurses to precept every novice. This is where the concept of multiple mentoring could be most effective. It allows novices and advanced beginners to seek out information from peers and competent nurses and then consult with proficient and expert nurses. Benner, Tanner, and Chesla (1996) found through their research that new nurses "know" what nurses are at what level very quickly after orientation, and so they know who to approach for particular needs. They found it takes approximately 2 years for a novice or advanced beginner to advance to competent status. Thus, it would be prudent for a unit to offer mentoring or precepting support to all nurses with less than 2 years of experience. The ideas Zachary (2000) has identified for program design could be organized using Benner's model.

Training sessions need to include discussions of learning theories on how individuals learn. Ideas from Dewey (1933), Rogers (1969), and Knowles (1984) are helpful for preceptors to review. Bloom's Taxonomy (Anderson, 1994) needs to be addressed so that mentors know how to discriminate among knowledge, comprehension, application, analysis, and synthesis when teaching and conducting evaluations. Examples of applying the Revised Bloom's Taxonomy in the clinical laboratory can be helpful for mentors and preceptors (Su, Osisek, & Starnes, 2005). Maslow's Hierarchy of Needs (1954) is important to include for preceptors to review rationales for prioritization. Evaluation methods need to be discussed, and tools that are both formative and summative need to be developed. Finally, legal and ethical issues need to be integrated into the training of both mentors and preceptors.

Classic Mentoring Model

Nolinske (1995) describes a one-to-one mentoring model that identifies the mentor as an expert nurse. Nolinske also identifies a multiple mentor experience model that allows the mentee to have access to several experienced, supportive persons. This multiple model is comparable to the following description of the primary and secondary mentor model. A primary mentor presented a total commitment to the mentee, but a secondary mentor was more of a temporary role modeling experience or preceptorship on the side. Nolinske recommends the following five strategies to use for mentorship development:

1. Determine the purpose for the mentorship.
2. Train mentors so they are aware of the goals of the program.
3. Orient mentees to the goals of the program.
4. Pair mentors and mentees, but let them set up their own mutually agreed-on rules. (The organization should set up general rules such as recommended duration, time, frequency of interaction, and an evaluation process for use by each pair.)
5. Ensure that each is entering the mentoring relationship voluntarily and that no one is being coerced to mentor or be a mentee.

These are several common steps in mentorship development. The literature suggests establishing a mentoring program as an effective way to recruit and retain nurses. Pontius (2001), a vice president of nursing at a large, urban hospital, recommends that RN mentors with the following qualifications be used: RNs with impeccable clinical skills, RNs who have been preceptors, full-time or part-time RNs, RNs not involved in any discipline process, and RNs approved by the director of the mentor program. This hospital developed the following responsibilities for each mentor:

• Mentor and coach a nursing student or nurse by discussing academic issues, clinical issues, ethical questions, and how to manage test anxiety.
• Assume the leadership role in contacting the student or nurse and setting up a schedule with the student.
• Establish a relationship that is comfortable for the student or nurse and is not intrusive.

The goal is to support the person as he or she becomes more comfortable with the role of a nurse. It does not matter what clinical rotation the student is in for his or her nursing program. The mentor remains consistent. Once the student graduates, a survey is sent to the mentor and graduate or nurse to identify program outcomes. This program recommends hosting a reception during National Nurses Week to recognize nurses and showcase the mentoring program. This has been a successful advertising method. Outcomes have been evaluated as excellent for both the mentee and mentor, as well as cost-effective for the organization.

Pinkerton (2003) describes a similar mentoring program to assist new graduates and increase retention. Staff nurses interested in mentoring volunteer and are interviewed by the hospital's mentoring committee. An RN who is accepted by the committee signs an agreement to accomplish the assigned tasks of the mentor role. This is an 18-month commitment. The mentee then chooses a mentor from the identified list of mentors. There are three 6-month components of the mentorship, and so far, there has been no attrition. Of those completing the program (both the mentor and mentee), all have had extremely positive remarks regarding the educational growth of mentee, increased self-confidence of mentee and staff, and the increased retention on RNs.

Grindel (2003) offers many more specifics for setting up formal manager mentorship programs and says it is essential that there be a site mentorship coordinator with a support team. The team then develops a plan for the future manager and for the mentors. Included in the plan are mentor selection processes, implementation of the mentor-mentee relationship, a process for follow-up by the site coordinator, training of mentors and mentees, and evaluation of effectiveness of the partnership.

McMaster University School of Nursing set up a mentoring program whereby interested baccalaureate nursing students are mentored by alumni. They found positive outcomes for both mentees (support and advice with career goals) and for mentors (reconnection with the alma mater and satisfaction in sharing their knowledge and experience) (Sword, Byrne, Drummond-Young, Harmer, & Rush, 2002).

Multiple Mentoring Model

Those who are involved in a formal mentoring connection can still develop relationships with other mentors or be in a multiple mentoring process. In order to meet specific needs of new employees, some organizations set up formal multiple mentoring programs in which junior employees can search for mentors who can best assist them in a variety of areas. Burlew (1991) sets out the components of a multiple mentoring model:

- Training mentor. This mentor assists the new worker to adjust to the organizational climate. The person can be assigned or informally paired with the new worker.
- Education mentor. This mentor provides information on career advancement. He or she also focuses on training the mentee for a specific job, helping with developing strong support groups for the mentee, making plans for the future, planning educational opportunities, and accessing new skills for advancement.

- Development mentor. This mentor helps the mentee develop his or her potential for the greatest growth and productivity for the organization. This mentor also helps the mentee accomplish self-actualization as described in Maslow's Hierarchy of Needs (1954).

This multiple mentoring model states that it covers all aspects of career advancement, psychosocial development, and role modeling. Actually the mentee can have experiences with various mentors in each category in order to get the most effective mentoring. There are several advantages for mentees who are involved in a multiple mentoring process:

- Less wasted time looking for the perfect mentor
- Advice from a number of people
- Increased chance of diverse mentoring by gender or culture if desired
- Increased possibility to obtain mentoring from the most famous mentor in the work setting since this individual will be available to more than just one mentee

Similarly, the organization also benefits from this multiple mentoring process, as do the mentors, since they spend less time mentoring if they are involved with several mentees versus just one. Mentors also do not have to have sole responsibility for a mentee; if the mentee fails, there will be more than one mentor held accountable. The biggest disadvantage in a multiple mentoring model is that it is possible for a mentee who is not doing satisfactory work to get lost and not be effectively mentored by any of the mentors.

Internships are generally for new graduates being hired to work as entry-level staff nurses in an agency. Specialty units such as critical care units, labor and delivery units, emergency departments, operating rooms, and postanesthesia care units tend to have longer, more detailed content classes and one-on-one time with the preceptor. Medical-surgical units have internships as well, and they tend to have limited classroom time and more one-on-one clinical precepted time for an average duration of 4 weeks. During this time, preceptees need to complete the competency-based orientation program for their designated unit.

Externships tend to be temporary summer employment for student nurses who are not internal to the hospital or home care system. The goal is to ultimately hire the best nursing students to work after their externship is completed. Many agencies offer these 12-week programs to recruit the students to work for them per diem during holidays, weekends, and vacations and then as full-time employees after graduation.

Peer Mentoring Model

Some people network constantly, so this process of peer mentoring may be in existence informally for some people much of their lives. Often, peer mentoring develops within a cohort of new graduates or between the current cadre of new graduates and the most recent new graduates who are now staff nurses with one year of experience. Peer mentoring is an excellent informal opportunity to form lasting networks that may endure over the course of these individuals' careers. The relationships established tend to become stronger if the individuals have similar developmental stages. There are disadvantages to peer mentoring, such as confidentiality and competition, whereby some individuals spend their time breaking the network's integrity in order to set up others to fail. This type of behavior is generally manifested by one or two of the mentees, so they are identified and asked to resign from the group. Their professional survival in that organization is not likely going to be successful, and generally they move from institution to institution.

There are also formal peer mentoring programs in which new employees or incoming students are paired off with a "big sister or brother," a senior employee or older student. These programs are voluntary and depend on whether the younger person takes advantage of the assigned person. The quality of these pairings is dependent on how seriously the experienced individual takes his or her responsibility. Most organizations seem to have models of this type of mentoring assignment, and they can also be generally found at Web sites. For example, the National Student Nurses Association (http://www.nsna.org) offers an excellent benefit with networking possibilities with other students and nursing leaders from across the country. It also has an excellent video on mentoring available for minimal cost. The National Student Nurses Association Leadership University (www.leadershipu. org) has information on setting up mentorships that can be downloaded. And the Nursing Net's mentoring project (www.nursingnet.org) allows a registered nurse to ask for a mentor with specific criteria or allows the individual to select a mentor. Finally, an online library that describes multiple mentoring programs is found at www.Questia.com.

Preceptorship Model

Flynn (1997) describes in her book, *The Role of the Preceptor: A Guide for Nurse Educators and Clinicians*, various strategies for setting up preceptor programs for nurses. She also describes two exemplary models: for a health teaching urban medical center and for a school of nursing. The book provides copies of orientation skill checklists, orientation curricula, evaluation tools, criteria for preceptor selection, policies for senior nursing students doing rotations with preceptors, and self-assessment forms for preceptees that can be modified for use in a variety of settings.

The precepting model is a one-on-one relationship in which the experienced nurse provides the preceptee with opportunities to practice, with supervision, working with the common patient types of the unit. The preceptor facilitates opportunities for the new employee to practice each skill delineated on a unit-developed skill checklist. A successful completion of skills and critical thinking situations allows the new nurse to complete orientation. Even after orientation, new nurses need coaching and further precepting when assigned to high-acuity, unstable patients with diseases they have not had any previous experience with certain skills such as intravenous insertion, specific medication administration protocols, codes, and any unit-specific procedures such as chronic ambulatory peritoneal dialysis or ventilator management that is skill intensive. If the preceptee is a student, the focus will be on accomplishing course objectives, not on mastery of all of the unit-specific skills and challenges.

It is extremely challenging for a staff nurse who is already overloaded to precept a nursing student who is not well prepared. Matsumura, Callister, Palmer, Cox, and Larson (2004) used Grindel's (2001) *Contributions of Students to Clinical Agencies Tool* to study staff nurse perceptions of students. The findings of the sample (N = 108, consisting of psychiatric and medical-surgical staff nurses) showed that staff nurses perceive definite benefits of having the students on their units as long as they are prepared and willing to help out with any task for any patient and not just their assigned one or two patients. Nurse faculty can have a strong impact on the success of students' rotation in any health care agency by providing them with an introduction to the unit and the organization to which they are assigned. Students need to have time to practice skills in the simulated laboratory, then advance to extended care facilities where they can become comfortable talking to and assisting patients with their activities of daily living, then to practicing total patient care and honing time management skills in subacute care facilities, then to hospitals, and finally to the patient's home. By gradually assuming more and more responsibility and having time to practice on less acutely ill patients initially, nursing students can gain confidence with their clinical, health teaching, and leadership and management skills prior to having rotations in hospitals and home care. Andrews and Wallis (1999) say that mentoring of students in England has become the responsibility of bedside nurses and not nurse educators. With fewer and fewer resources being available in academia and clinical services, there is often little preparation of preceptors.

Models for preceptoring programs are set up for new graduates, senior- and junior-year nursing students, and the transition of RNs to new clinical areas and RN retraining. A step or phase framework is not generally used. Rather, preceptorships are developed as one-on-one assignments in order to allow the preceptee time to gain specific experience. Often due to RN schedules, students have more than one preceptor to whom they are assigned to work with during a rotation. There is, however, more of a trend today to have a student follow the RN's schedule in order to provide preceptor consistency for the student. RNs orienting with a staff nurse preceptor generally have a consistent preceptor they are assigned to work on the shift they were hired for after completing approximately 1–2 days of general agency and unit orientation.

One nurse mentoring program was started due to low retention of RNs: 21 nurses had terminated their employment within 18 months of hire. The program was started with these for underlying goals (Greene & Puetzer, 2002):

1. Develop and maintain relationships between new and current staff.
2. Promote team building.
3. Guide novice nurses in the culture and environment of the new role.
4. Recognize and use clinical experts currently on staff. (A mentor was defined as an experienced and competent staff nurse who serves as a role model and resource person to an assigned new staff member. The mentor must commit to a one-year relationship.)

The mentee was defined as a newly hired staff nurse participating in the orientation program. Due to time constraints and the orientation timetable, assigned pairings were used. A mentor was defined as a role model, a socializer, and an educator. As a role model, the mentor assists the mentee by example, that is, demonstrating how a competent staff nurse performs the job; as a socializer, the mentor integrates the mentee into the social culture of the unit and facility; as an educator, the mentor assists the mentee in planning his or her orientation. The mentee must be open to feedback, know his or her goals and work to accomplish them, have career commitment and competence, and demonstrate a strong self-identity and initiative. This model is developed in collaboration with the nursing process:

1. Assessment. Make time to get to know each other, develop goals, and review the time frame and expectations. Review the competency behavior checklist.

2. Planning. Choose assignments carefully to allow for goal achievement as well as long- and short-term planning.
3. Implementation. Demonstrate knowledge through course work and use of current policy and the procedure book. Use a variety of methods so attitudes can be shaped through role playing, case study review, value clarification, and discussions. Practice skills are done in a simulation laboratory and also include critical thinking exercises.
4. Evaluation. The preceptee must demonstrate evaluation skills with charting of data collection, analysis, planning, implementation, and outcome management.

Mentors receive the following incentives: wage adjustment, flexibility of scheduling, and title recognition (Santos & Cox, 2002).

Meno, Keaveny, and O'Donnell (2003) present the perceptions of student nurse anesthetists ($N = 1,251$) on mentoring in the clinical setting and offer suggestions for developing a mentoring model for this type of student. The study identified the most important mentor traits to include: being knowledgeable, approachable, encouraging, and a practicing Certified Registered Nurse Anesthetist (CRNA). Hand and Thompson (2003) conducted a study of nurses anesthesia preceptors ($N = 90$) to determine their perceptions of mentoring and if they felt they were actually mentoring the students they precepted. The majority agreed that they were mentoring the students, felt the students perceived they were mentoring them, and valued mentoring the students. Seventy-nine percent had had mentors during their educational program and felt they had had multiple mentors in their careers. Mentoring seemed to be confused with precepting in most cases, but a few had experienced a long-term mentoring relationship with either an anesthesiologist or nurse anesthetist. The authors question if it is feasible for every anesthesia student to have a mentor and suggest that it is the precepting that really counts. They advocate that faculty spend more time developing clinical preceptors to be more mentoring than trying to be a mentor to every student. In fact, they say it is important for the educators to be supportive to all but not feasible to be a mentor to every student. This finding is significant for all practicum-intensive graduate programs.

Hayes (1998) discusses factors that increase self-efficacy as well as mentoring scores for nurse practitioner students. She found that nurse practitioner students do better with self-efficacy scores if they can choose their own mentor. This was particularly true if the student had a current relationship with the nurse practitioner. This information is particularly helpful for nurse practitioner program directors who may be having a difficult time obtaining preceptors. Acquiring preceptors is a labor-intensive process, so if outcomes are more positive if students obtain their own preceptors, it may be a win-win situation. Perhaps the preceptors may be more mentoring if they are approached by a student than a faculty member. The nurse practitioner directors can spend this time more effectively by teaching other aspects of the nurse practitioner role such as research, consultation, counseling, teaching, quality assurance, case management, and influencing health policy. Studies conducted in the late 1980s and early 1990s (Freeman, 1989; Thibodeau & Hawkins, 1994) found that many nurse practitioner students do not get socialized into the multifaceted nurse practitioner role since the preceptor tends to be focused solely on direct patient care.

Shadowing Model

Shadowing is a process by which a less experienced individual shadows or follows an experienced individual through a component of the day's work. The person shadowing is not expected to fulfill work at the workplace of the person being shadowed. The focus is strictly an observational experience. Prospective RN candidates sometimes choose to shadow a nurse for 4 hours or so prior to accepting a position on a unit. There are also many programs that link a person interested in a nursing career to shadow a nurse for a few hours. The nursing student shadowee has objectives for each shadowing experience that are mutually reviewed and agreed on with the person being shadowed. This is generally a process used with students, so there are also general goals for the shadowee to accomplish with the experience in order to complete the course objectives.

Grossman (2005) reports about senior students in their leadership and management rotation being assigned to shadow a leader in health care for a semester. They were paired with an individual in one of the following areas (students did choose the area and when possible, although rarely, chose the mentor): patient advocacy, health education, research, quality improvement, health care policy, and hospital/home care administration. By engaging in supervised leadership activities such as negotiating conflicts, participating in collaborative decision making, assisting in health policy development and medical compliance assessments, and creating clinical and patient education protocols, students were able to experience practicing leadership firsthand during the daily activities of a health care leader. Students' leadership development scores as measured by the Grossman and Valiga Leadership Characteristics and Skills Assessment (Grossman & Valiga, 2005) were statistically significantly higher after the experience.

Students kept logs and in their final assessment described their leadership growth:

"I have consciously begun to acknowledge the fear that I have as a new graduate, am able to conduct an internal dialogue with myself about the fear, and attempt to conquer the apprehension I have so that I can start to work on a specific goal."

"I think that if I were to develop more reliability and that if I could actively practice being more accountable I will become more competent and receive more respect for what I do."

"I've learned to be more enthusiastic in order to be persuasive and get people to understand and accept a plan."

"It has become clear to me that my reluctance to trust others to get important tasks done right has a lot to do with patience, I am less apt to hover annoyingly around people as they work and I also butt in and make suggestions less often now and I certainly no longer insist on doing everything myself!"

Students demonstrated this growth after shadowing their mentor for a semester. The following themes were identified after reviewing three logs for each student:

- Growth over the semester specifically regarding increased self-confidence with communication skills
- Greater interest in becoming politically astute and aware of the importance of the organizational culture of the mentor's agency
- Improved awareness of the benefits of partnering, collaborating, and networking
- Awareness of the importance of learning negotiation and conflict management skills

These themes are similar to what Glass (1998) identified as comprising the empowerment of nurses: raised consciousness, strong self-esteem, and political skills have an impact on the health care system. Nurses need to cultivate these skills to be change agents.

Mentees were excited about their mentors and shared descriptions of them—for example:

"He was able to get everyone on board with the change he was about to implement about staffing the step-down unit."

"It was really exceptional working right alongside the CEO of the agency and being a part of the decisions—she really valued my input."

"My mentor made this experience one of the best that I have had because he made me believe in myself."

"My mentor showed me how to delegate and how essential this is to my overall productivity and sense of accomplishment" (Grossman, 2005).

It seems this mentorship helped to empower students to become more autonomous and accountable in their own right regarding leadership skills.

Coaching Model

Coaching does not involve the formality of a mentorship or preceptorship. It is advice given to others generally on a regular basis but can be limited to even a one-time experience in order to assist a less experienced individual in accomplishing a goal. The goals are not developed with the coach; they are strictly the learner's. In fact, the learner's goals may not even be known to the coach. Generally the less experienced individual seeks counsel from a more experienced nurse, who then acts as a coach regarding troubleshooting complex equipment, analyzing laboratory or physical assessment data, or assisting the nurse to decide if a patient's condition is deteriorating. There are no data evaluating this process, nor does it tend to be sponsored through an organization. What transpires is generally spontaneous in that an inexperienced nurse seeks help from an experienced nurse. There are, however, coaching programs developing in clinical practice for nurses that are sponsored by the workplace. Coaching is, in essence, coming back, or at least it is in nursing. Many hospitals have set up support systems for the nursing staff using clinical resource nurses or clinical nurse specialists. These nurses do not have a patient assignment but instead are assigned to certain units on a specified shift to make rounds and assist nurses with their needs. Nurses also have the option of calling this individual to assist them with a challenging, unstable patient or help them with a procedure or admission or transfer. Although mentoring is differentiated between coaching (a senior staff member teaches a skill to assigned junior staff in a limited time frame) and precepting (an assigned, seasoned staff member orients and trains a new employee for the first few weeks of being hired), there are many similarities. Certainly after precepting or coaching, it is possible for a mentoring bond to develop spontaneously and evolve over a longer period of time. In this way, the preceptor or coach shares the responsibility the mentor has to the mentee, which is to teach the mentee the ropes but also to share "the untold story, which is not always about the obvious workings of the job, but how the job really gets done." This "perpetual essence" of mentoring is the shaping of the mentee to create another mentor or preceptor or coach for the future (Fox & Shephard, 1998, p. 153).

Role Modeling

Role modeling is a process by which a less experienced individual chooses a person he or she wishes to emulate. This is often done from afar, and the role model is not even aware of the other individual.

Mentoring Partnerships

Nickitas, Keida, Nokes, and Neville (2004) discuss using the service-learning approach in planning practica for nursing administration students. They used the principles of partnership as described by Seifer (2002) to assist them in developing these rotations. Academia has used this model in which a nursing student is paired up with a patient recently discharged or in need of health teaching in the community who also is mentored by a counselor, nurse, or some other type of health care worker at a health care agency in the community. It is also used for nurses working in hospitals who are coming back for an advanced degree and may be paired with an undergraduate student in the same school of nursing. This partnering assists the RN, the nursing student, the health care agency recruitment initiative, and the school of nursing. With the nursing shortage, there probably will be more use of nursing students to extend nursing to needed individuals, and this can be delivered under a partnership program. In this way, the hospital, the nurses, the students, the school of nursing, and, most important, the patients will all enjoy a win-win situation.

An excellent example of partnering nursing students and RNs at health care agencies occurred with a college of nursing and two community hospitals. Students were told about the program and asked to volunteer to attend a luncheon to meet potential mentors. Nursing faculty were not involved in this partnership except for the initial announcements explaining the program. Rather, the program encourages mentors and mentees to interact at the luncheon and determine their own mentoring or shadowing relationship. What ensues is completely between the nurses and the students (McCadden, 2003). This two-way learning process generated outcomes including extremely satisfied nursing students and RN mentors feeling a growth of new nursing ideas from the students.

Anderson, Richmond, and Stanhope (2004) developed a collaborative partnership between the Kentucky Department of Public Health and University of Kentucky College of Nursing in order to

- strengthen the public health nursing practice component of the nursing program;
- offer students a broader public health rotation;
- afford the student exposure to work in practice with a public health nurse and also in policy development at the local or state level.

No outcome measurement was offered, but trends indicate positive responses on the public health and policy development components.

Paper Mentorships

There are many nursing journals that give accounts of how a nurse mentored new staff, students, or peers. For example, Fox and Shephard (1998) emphasize the importance for mentors and mentees to share their experiences in the editorial column of the *Journal of Neuroscience Nursing*. This helps others to go out and develop a mentorship by reading others' stories. Most of these accounts include some advice to the reader on how to and how not to do certain things related to career development and getting acclimated to a new job. One resource that is helpful for nurses to use in answering frequently asked questions regarding mentoring others is *What Color Is Your Parachute?* (Bolles, 1999). Although paper mentoring is not traditional mentoring, it does serve to fulfill some needs of individuals new to an organization or career and can act as a supplement.

MULTICULTURAL COMPETENCY IN MENTORING

That there is a separate component of this chapter on multicultural competence speaks to the nonintegration of cultural competency in the majority of mentoring models. Most preceptors are not of the same culture as their preceptee, so it is of utmost importance to have the preceptors trained in cultural competency. Actually, all nurses and health care workers should be trained, and there should be multiple strategies to heighten awareness. Some mentors and mentees may be from the same culture but have very different levels of cultural sensitivity. Coffman, Shellman, and Bernal (2004) suggest that nurses lack cultural self-efficacy, information, and experience with culturally diverse groups. Cultural stereotypes for Asian Americans,

Hispanic Americans, and African Americans need to be discussed, and perhaps, doing role-plays of some of these issues will increase awareness among preceptors so they do not show prejudice to their preceptees.

It is critically important for all nurses to be educated to identify and manage issues of culture in the work setting. With the multidiverse population today nurses need to be culturally aware. The American Association of Colleges of Pharmacy and Association of American Medical Colleges co-hosted a webcast, "Cultural Competence in Health-Professions Training: Considerations for Implementation," on May 12, 2005. The objectives for this program included discussion of the underpinnings, benefits, and challenges of building a culturally competent health professions workforce; increasing knowledge about two approaches being used to implement and assess cultural competence training; and learning about resources to improve efforts to integrate cultural competence training. There was a $100 fee per site for a live performance for as many health care professionals who desired to attend the site. Each professional attending received a CD-ROM version of the program.

It is paramount that preceptors be taught about learning styles and professional practice of nursing of various cultures. Frusti, Niesen, and Campion (2003) developed a mentoring model including all types of diversity, including gender, race, culture, disability, and religion, to increase awareness for health care staff. It is imperative that all nurses be aware of the career and educational resources available today in most health care settings. Leaders need to assess their organization's readiness to respond to diversity initiatives. The diversity competency model includes leadership commitment, structural links, organizational culture, and continuous measurements to assess the success of the mentorship from both the mentee and mentor's perspectives. Preceptees, especially nurses from other countries on travel contracts, need to be socialized to the culture of America and that of the health care agency. Characteristics of intercultural mentoring are shared with specific strategies to improve student cultural competency by Koskinen and Tossavainen (2003). Murrell, Crosby, and Ely (1999) suggest multiple strategies for reflecting diversity in mentoring programs. They share experiences in business and educational organizations regarding dilemmas that mentors and mentees face. They demonstrate how theory and practice must be integrated into a mentoring program in order to meet diverse needs. Green-Hernandez, Quinn, Deman-Vitale, Falkenstern, and Judge-Ellis (2004) offer insights into cultural diversity in primary care that are helpful for mentors and mentees in any setting. Zachary (2000) provides many cross-cultural mentoring strategies that can be revised and used in any work setting:

- Reflective listening
- Checking for understanding
- Maintaining cultural self-awareness
- Providing and receiving feedback
- Maintaining a global perspective
- Suspending judgment
- Maintaining emotional versatility
- Exercising cultural flexibility
- Creating culturally appropriate networking opportunities
- Modifying communication style to accommodate cultural differences
- Sensitivity to varying cultural perceptions to time, space, authority, and protocol

Johnson and Huwe (2003) believe there must be structured mentoring programs for minority group students, especially if the campus is predominantly one culture. Some of the components they suggest are assignment of a faculty mentor and peer adviser, entry into an established student support network, and planned workshops to prepare students for various aspects of the graduate program in which they are enrolled. They recognize that intentionally assigning mentee to mentor is not the traditional mentoring method but feel it is necessary to have culturally aware or similar matches as well as experienced mentors working with minority students. Boyd (2002) speaks to "mentoring at the margin," meaning that there are benefits and risks of working with students of marginalized status.

Some successful programs with planned mentorships such as this include Peabody Mentoring Program at Vanderbilt University; the Graduate Mentorship Program at the University of California, Berkeley; the Graduate Opportunities and Minority Achievement Program at the University of Washington; and the Coordinating Council for Minority Issues at the University of Chicago. Nugent, Childs, Jones, and Cook (2004) developed the Mentorship Model for the Retention of Minority Students to assist students with academic support, self-development, financial support, and professional leadership development. Outcomes from using their model proved to be positive for retaining minority students and increasing their leadership skills.

CONCLUSION

It seems that the ideal mentoring and precepting model would have to be both informally and formally assigned with traditional mentoring connections.

Multiple mentoring models appear to be the most appropriate option for new nurses in all areas of clinical practice. The classic mentoring process is most appropriate for the doctoral student or new faculty member who needs long-term mentoring in order to be successful. Peer mentoring models are informal networks that assist all individuals to gain benefits. One-size mentoring programs do not exist. There needs to be individualization depending on the mentee's and organization's needs. More research is needed on how best to provide cultural competency in mentoring models. The idea of having several mentors in an individual's career seems to be most effective. Alliances with a mentor may develop in various ways over one's adult life, both professionally and personally. Effective mentoring increases productivity and adds to a more collegial relationship. The profession has a long road to go before the mentoring culture will be evident in all settings.

REFERENCES

Anderson, D., Richmond, C., & Stanhope, M. (2004). Enhanced undergraduate public health nursing experience: A collaborative experience with the Kentucky Department of Public Health. *Family and Community Health, 27,* 291–297.

Anderson, L. (1994). *Bloom's taxonomy: A forty-year retrospective.* New York: NSSE.

Andrews, M., & Wallis, M. (1999). Mentorship in nursing: A literature review. *Journal of Advanced Nursing, 29,* 201–207

Benner, P. (1984). *From novice to expert: Excellence and power in clinical nursing practice.* Menlo Park, CA: Addison-Wesley.

Benner, P., Tanner, C., & Chesla, C. (1996). *Expertise in nursing practice: Caring, clinical judgment, and ethics.* New York: Springer Publishing.

Bennetts, C. (2000). The traditional mentor relationship and the well-being of creative individuals in school and work. *International Journal of Health Promotion and Education, 38,* 22–27.

Bolles, R. (1999). *What color is your parachute?* Berkeley, CA: Ten Speed Press.

Bower, F. (2000). *Nurses taking the lead: Personal qualities of effective leadership.* Philadelphia: W. B. Saunders.

Boyd, N. (2002). Mentoring dilemmas: Developmental relationships within multicultural organizations. *Journal of Occupational and Organizational Psychology, 75,* 123–126.

Burlew, L. (1991). Multiple mentor model: A conceptual framework. *Journal of Career Development, 17,* 213–221.

Byrne, M., & Keefe, M. (2003). A mentored experience (K01) in maternal—infant research. *Journal of Professional Nursing, 19,* 66–75.

Coffman, M., Shellman, J., & Bernal, H. (2004). An integrative review of American nurses' perceived cultural self-efficacy. *Journal of Nursing Scholarship, 36,* 180–185.

Dewey, J. (1933). *How we teach: A restatement of the relation of reflective thinking to the education process.* Boston: Heath.

Flynn, J. P. (1997). *The role of the preceptor: A guide for nurse educators and clinicians.* New York: Springer Publishing.

Fox, S., & Shephard, T. (1998). The essence of mentoring. *Journal of Neuroscience Nursing, 30,* 1–3.

Freeman, S. (1989). The mentor experience as perceived by nurse practitioners: Implications for curriculum design. (Doctoral dissertation, Georgia State University, 1989). *Dissertation Abstracts International, 51,* 22–44.

Frusti, D., Niesen, K., & Campion, J. (2003). Creating a culturally competent organization: Use of the diversity competency model. *Journal of Nursing Administration, 33,* 31–38.

Glass, N. (1998). Becoming de-silenced and reclaiming voice: Women nurses speak out. In I. Kelleher & P. McInerney (Eds.), *Nursing matters* (pp. 127–137). Melbourne, Australia: Harcourt Brace.

Green-Hernandez, C., Quinn, A., Deman-Vitale, S., Falkenstern, S., & Judge-Ellis, T. (2004). Making primary care culturally competent. *Nurse Practitioner, 29,* 49–55.

Greene, M., & Puetzer, M. (2002). The value of mentoring: A strategic approach to retention and recruitment. *Journal of Nursing Care Quality, 17,* 67–74.

Grindel, C. (2003). Mentoring managers. *Nephrology Nursing Journal, 30,* 517–522.

Grossman, S. (2005). Developing leadership through shadowing a leader in health care. In H. Feldman & M. Greenberg (Eds.), *Educating nurses for leadership* (pp. 266–278). New York: Springer Publishing.

Grossman, S., & Valiga, T. (2005). *The new leadership challenge: Creating the future of nursing* (2nd ed.). Philadelphia: F. A. Davis.

Hand, R., & Thompson, E. (2003). Are we really mentoring our students? *American Association of Nurse Anesthesia Journal, 71,* 105–108.

Hayes, E. F. (1998). Mentoring and nurse practitioner student self-efficacy. *Western Journal of Nursing Research, 20,* 521–535.

Johnson, W., & Huwe, J. (2003). *Getting mentored: In graduate school.* Washington, DC: American Psychological Association.

Knowles, M. (1984). *Andragogy in action: Applying modern principles of adult learning.* San Francisco: Jossey-Bass.

Kosikinen, L., & Tossavainen, K. (2003). Characteristics of intercultural mentoring: A mentor perspective. *Nurse Education Today, 23,* 278–285.

Kram, K. (1983). Phases of the mentor relationship. *Academy of Management Journal, 26,* 608–625.

Luna, G., & Cullen, D. (1996). *Empowering the faculty: Mentoring redirected and renewed.* Washington, DC: George Washington University Press.

Maslow, A. (1954). *Motivation and personality.* New York: Harper & Row.

Matsumura, G., Callister, L., Palmer, S., Cox, A., & Larsen, L. (2004). Staff nurse perceptions of the contributions of students to clinical agencies. *Nursing Education Perspectives, 25,* 297–303.

McCadden, L. (2003). Perfect partnerships: Mentor program lets nursing students and professional learn from one another. *Advance for Nurses, New England, 9,* 23, 38.

Meno, K., Keaveny, B., & O'Donnell, J. (2003). Mentoring in the operating room, a student perspective. *AANA Journal, 71,* 337–341.

Murrell, A., Crosby, F., & Ely, R. (1999). *Mentoring dilemmas: Developmental relationships within multicultural organizations.* Hillside, NJ: Erlbaum.

Nickitas, D., Keida, R., Nokes, K., & Neville, S. (2004). Nurturing nursing future through nurse executive partnerships. *Nursing Economics, 22,* 258–263.

Nolinske, T. (1995). Multiple mentoring relationships facilitate learning during fieldwork. *American Journal of Occupational Therapy, 49,* 39–43.

Nugent, K., Childs, G., Jones, R., & Cook, P. (2004). A mentorship model for the retention of minority students. *Nursing Outlook, 52,* 89–94.

Pinkerton, S. (2003). Mentoring new graduates. *Nursing Economics, 2,* 202–203.

Pontius, C. (2001). Meant to be a mentor. *Nursing Management, 32,* 35.

Rogers, C. (1969). *Freedom to learn: A view of what education might become.* New York: C. E. Merrill.

Santos, S., & Cox, K. (2002). Generational tension among nurses. *American Journal of Nursing, 102*(1), 11.

Schwiebert, N. (2000). *Mentoring: Creating connected, empowered relationships.* Alexandria, VA: American Counseling Association.

Seifer, S. (2002). From placement site to partnership: The promise of service learning. *Journal of Nursing Education, 41,* 431–432.

Senge, P., Kleiner, A., Roberts, C., Ross, R., & Smith, B. (1994). *The fifth discipline fieldbook: Strategies and tools for building a learning organization.* New York: Doubleday.

Senge, P., Scharmer, C., Jaworski, J., & Flowers, B. (2004). *Presence: Human purpose and the field of the future.* Cambridge, MA: Society for Organizational Learning.

Smith, L., McAllister, L., & Crawford, C. (2001). Mentoring benefits and issues for public health nurses. *Public Health Nursing, 18,* 101–107.

Snell, J. (1999). Mentoring: Head to head. *Health Services Journal, 109,* 22–25.

Su, W., Osisek, P., & Starnes, B. (2005). Using the revised Bloom's taxonomy in the clinical laboratory: Learning, teaching, and assessing. *Nurse Educator, 30,* 117–122.

Sword, W., Byrne, C., Drummond-Young, M., Harmer, M., & Rush, J.(2002). Nursing alumni as student mentors: Nurturing professional growth. *Nurse Education Today, 22,* 427–432.

Thibodeau, J., & Hawkins, J. (1994). Moving toward a nursing model in advanced practice. *Western Journal of Nursing Research, 16,* 205–218.

Zachary, L. (2000). *The mentor's guide: Facilitating effective learning relationships.* San Francisco: Jossey Bass.

CHAPTER 5

The Mentor Perspective on How Best to Encourage Others

$\mathbf{M}$yrick (2002) found that "preceptors were more likely to enable critical thinking indirectly through their role modeling, facilitating, guiding, and prioritizing than they were to directly influence preceptees' critical thinking through questioning" (p. 161). Preceptors can role-model leadership for new nurses and students and facilitate opportunities for them to practice leadership just as they practice calibrating a pulmonary artery catheter or interpreting a telemetry strip.

Much regarding the future of the profession of nursing depends on those who are mentoring nurses—the preceptors, coaches, role models, and mentors. Some are people in authority, others are peers, some are nurses, and some are from other disciplines. But all are leaders, and they are cognizant that leadership is not a position or a skill but a relationship (Kouzes & Posner, 1993). Most have a great amount of wisdom to pass to others. Sullivan (2004) reminds us that when discussing mentoring, the question is not, "What is it?" but rather, "What can it be?" Today, with such transitional times in health care, it is essential for mentors to

- foster optimism and hope for the future;
- be strong leaders who role-model how nurses cannot be compliant and fit in with the current system;
- communicate that nurses can and do make a huge difference.

Block (1996) has good advice for mentors: tell the truth and have integrity above all else, show passion for one's work, know what is important for oneself, and take responsibility for one's own life. He recommends that it is best not to fragmentize one's life into compartments such as spiritual, private and personal, and work and professional. Rather, he suggests trying to live without always planning every step, following every good career and professional move, and not having to always be in control of those around us. In his book *Stewardship: Choosing Service Over Self-Interest*, he recommends that leaders not try to help mentees define their purpose and meaning, but rather let them do this entirely themselves, even if they ask for help. Block provides ways to find partnerships and be who you want to be, and suggests how to become and remain empowered.

This chapter describes methods for capturing the role of an effective mentor; delineates characteristics of effective mentors, preceptors, and coaches; and identifies benefits for those who participate in some form of mentoring.

ROLE OF THE EFFECTIVE MENTOR, PRECEPTOR, OR COACH

Most significant to a successful mentorship is having an effective mentor who possesses the following characteristics: has excellent communication skills, is approachable and flexible, is willing to put time into the relationship to give frequent feedback, is passionate about mentoring, and has good connections to assist with the mentee's career success (Andrews & Wallis, 1999; McCall, 1998). Others (Kram, 1983; Luna & Cullen, 1996 Shea, 1999; Sinetar, 1998;) add that it is also vital for organizations to specifically identify their goals of the mentorship and for mentors and mentees to develop contracts that are mutually satisfying to the mentee, mentor, and the organization. The contract should build on the mentee's and mentor's strengths as well as the mentor's resources and take into consideration any limitations of the relationship. A contract between a mentor and mentee should contain the specific time commitment, frequency of meeting, expected mentor role (coach, advisor, teacher), short- and long-term goals, and method of evaluation with target evaluation dates. Johnson and Huwe (2003) provide an example of a contract that could be revised for use by any mentor-mentee dyad.

Stone (1999) adds that mentors need to advocate for their mentees to attempt to maintain their motivation and also to keep aware of all potential opportunities that could be useful for mentees to use their talents so that maximum benefit can be obtained. These suggestions can assist mentors to do the following:

- Gather information. The mentor always needs to be assessing the mentee, without being unnecessarily interrogative, in order to be able to identify any deficiencies, confusion regarding the job, or problems. The mentor needs to redesign the contract plan to manage these concerns.

- Listen. It is imperative to hear all of the information and ask relevant questions when necessary. Be astute to nonverbal communications as well.
- Be aware of the workplace milieu. Know what the grassroots are talking about, correct any rumors, maintain a positive sense, and stay connected to the mentee.
- Be knowledgeable of work. Be competent with whatever work the mentee is involved in.
- Evaluate. Be able to give both positive and constructive feedback. Coach the mentee in finding solutions to problems in order to accomplish goals.

Bell (2002) proposes using the Surrendering/Accepting/Gifting/Extending (SAGE) Model for describing the role of a mentor:

- Surrendering. There is sometimes a need to level the playing field to foster more open discussion between mentor and mentee and to remove the power and authority from the mentoring relationship. Any anxiety that power creates should be eliminated in order to create an open environment.
- Accepting. Most frequently a mentor will have some degree of bias or preconceived judgments of the mentee. It is imperative that the mentor embraces the mentee for who the person really is so that open dialogue can transpire.
- Gifting. Mentors must be willing to share their passion for their work with the mentee. By advising and providing feedback, focus, and direction, mentors extend their passion for learning.
- Extending. Mentors need to push the mentee to stretch for the highest goals and constantly challenge the mentee to go beyond his or her expected goals.

Bell and Ross, Wenzel, and Mitlyng (2002) advise that mentors have skills in facilitating, guiding, encouraging, coaching, managing conflict, problem solving, providing and receiving feedback, reflecting, building and maintaining relationships, and goal setting in order to fulfill the mentor role. Lowney (2003) says what separates winning mentors from losing mentors is *leadership*.

Other recommendations come from Gilley and Boughton (1996), who advocate 10 steps to create a successful mentoring relationship:

1. Create a network.
2. Allow freedom.
3. Invest time wisely.
4. Be willing to give to receive.
5. Develop patience.
6. Actively listen to increase the effectiveness of the relationship.
7. Hopefully have chemistry with the mentee.
8. Establish relationship boundaries.
9. Create relationship reciprocity, and be aware the mentee may advance beyond you.
10. Develop synergy.

Certainly having a network that a mentee can become part of will be extremely advantageous for accomplishing the mentee's goals and strengthening one's own connections. It is imperative to have a mentee with true potential in order to even want to invest any time in a relationship. By believing in the mentee and giving freedom for the mentee to follow his or her own ideas, mentors empower the mentees to be successful with their work. A mentor must have the patience not to interfere and allow the mentee to figure out issues. A good chemistry between mentor and mentee adds to the possibilities of having a reciprocal, synergistic, give-and-take relationship in which both mentor and mentee open doors for each other. Levinson, Darrow, Klein, Levinson, and McKee (1978) echo these recommendations. As the initial writers and researchers about mentoring, Levinson et al. identified the mentor's functions to include

- sponsoring entry and advancement for the mentee;
- providing skills and knowledge;
- guiding the mentee through complex occupational and social paths;
- inculcating cultural and organizational values and customs.

It is desirable for the mentor and mentee to share similar philosophies of work, have even-tempered personalities, be flexible so as to be successful in seizing opportunities when they present, and possess similar ideas regarding the balance of professional and personal life.

Mentors need to fuel the mentee's enthusiasm as well as coach this person to pursue his or her goals (Zey, 1990; Ross et al., 2002). Mentors know they will learn from new employees who come with a fresh knowledge base, energy, and, in some cases, their own networks from graduate school or previous employment. Good mentors also know that even mentors need mentoring, and they must continue to build and rely on lifelong contacts who share their expertise. They must have a genuine and overriding interest in the business of developing people. Mentors need to teach and role-model how to network, develop outside partnerships, and prevent isolation or "becoming silos" with little connection to the outside world. By building from the inside out in organizations, shared governance facilitates employees to have more of a voice in the system and to include themselves more in developing outside connections. An effective mentor can role-model anticipating what could happen before it happens (Watkins & Bazerman, 2003).

It is important to realize mentors not only give but receive. McFarland, Senn, and Childress (1994) point out multiple ways for mentors to become part of an initiative or change that might have been originally developed for the mentee. Good mentors know there is more than enough room for the mentor to participate as well. Some mentors counsel their mentees to have two mentors: one in the same organization as the mentee and one outside the organization to provide different perspectives about work environments. It is only with partnering with others, sometimes even with groups or individuals who do not appear to be strong contributors, that true growth and success will occur. By mentoring others, success will be accomplished. It really is not possible to succeed as an individual; we must go out and partner.

Other suggestions in the literature include not taking over mentee problems and trying to solve them and not giving advice and solutions. Mentors who do this will only enable their mentees and prevent them from becoming empowered. Shea (1999) presents a method of assessing one's ability to communicate with his tool, Evaluating Your Communication Habits. Mentors can determine their own skills and their mentees with this assessment. Everyone needs to develop good communication skills in order to be sure their message is being received correctly. Gilley and Boughton (1996, p. 76) relate an interesting story regarding poor communication: The stewardess notes the right engine is on fire and calls the cockpit and tells the pilot who quickly shuts off the right engine. The plane crashes and burns . . . what happened? The stewardess and pilot were facing in different directions so that the stewardess's right side of the plane was the pilot's left side. This example is very effective in demonstrating how significant it is to be accurate and articulate clearly. Miscommunications do not often lead to a plane crash but can lead to multiple problems.

Robinson-Walker (1999) reports from her research with approximately 100 health care leaders that to be successful, one needs to tolerate ambiguity, be collaborative, demonstrate integrity, be able to negotiate fluently, and build consensus among a group. Lanser (2000) says a mentor must establish trust with the mentee to have a successful relationship. This is very true and is part of what Kouzes and Posner (1993) talk about when they say leaders must be credible. Their study included surveying 15,000 people, interpreting 400 case studies, and conducting 40 in-depth interviews regarding what constituents expect from leaders. They found the top four qualities leaders should possess: honesty, competence, forward looking, and inspiring. These four characteristics equal credibility. They suggest the three cornerstones of credibility: clarity, intensity, and unity. From this foundation Kouzes and Posner developed a framework of six methods to strengthen one's credibility. A mentor definitely needs to be credible in order to foster a favorable mentoring relationship. Kouzes and Posner advocate that mentor-leaders follow the Six Disciplines of Credibility:

1. Discovering yourself. Review with yourself who you are. What do you stand for? What do you believe in? After establishing standards by which to live your life, it will be easier to make decisions and develop your character—that is, your credo, competence, and confidence.
2. Appreciating constituents. Determine the values and desires of your constituents, and engage in dialogue with them. Be present, and listen to them. Always seek diversity of views, and look at the whole picture. This will make you more flexible.
3. Affirming shared values. Determine a common ground for all to share. Unite people through a collaborative leadership style. Renew your community by having frequent forums on topics of interest to all.
4. Developing capacity. Be sure to develop continuously the capacity of each constituent so that people are skilled to do successful work. Keep people informed, and encourage risks so that maximum learning and outcomes will transpire.
5. Serving a purpose. Leaders must be other-serving, not self-serving. Demonstrate your commitment to the community.
6. Sustaining hope. During transitional times especially, keep hope alive. This will lead to more challenging achievements as well as goal accomplishment.

Reardon (2004) discusses the language of negotiation and makes several recommendations for gaining this skill. Mentors can assist mentees to improve and expand on their negotiation skills by modeling how to frame issues, develop specific communication strategies, and engage in successful-cross cultural persuasion.

Many have said the best way to be a good mentor is to have been a mentee. But the question that arises is, "Is this assuming that one had a good mentor?" Not necessarily. It is possible to learn to be a good mentor even though one had a poor mentor or even no mentor. Most believe that mentoring can be taught or at least role-modeled (Werner, 2002). A great amount of what makes a good mentor depends on the person's value system. For example, Werner, a retired nurse academician and hospital administrator, shares that she frequently used to ask candidates who were interviewing for positions or promotions, or prospective students, "Tell me about the very best nurse you have ever known," in order to determine the candidate's value system. She conversed with them regarding their previous mentoring and any role models they may have had in their past. She inquired how they viewed their accomplishments—solely as a result of their own hard work or due to collaborating with others. The answers revealed significant information about the person. Werner points out that it is not what the mentor sees, does, and says; it is more who the mentor is. It is traits such as strength, courage, independence, and ability to see potential in others that make a mentor effective.

Cohen's (1999) workable model, the Mentoring Model of Active Learning, assists mentors in being most effective in the mentoring relationship. This model has six dimensions:

1. Relationship. The mentor provides empathy, open-ended questions for dialogue, descriptive feedback, perception checks, and nonjudgmental responses.
2. Informative. The mentor assists the mentee to assess his or her job, review job history, require concrete answers, ask for solutions to problems, ensure accuracy, and rely on facts for decision making.
3. Facilitative. The mentor helps the mentee expand on viewpoints, provide information, analyze decisions with multiple viewpoints, reinforce commitment to goal achievement, learn the basis for current pursuits, and review career options.
4. Confrontative. The mentor assists the mentee with assessment of readiness, expression of concern for criticism, self-assessment of goals, proposed strategies for change, and belief in one's growth.
5. Mentor model. The mentor role-models for the mentee how to learn from difficulty, be motivated and be committed to plan, while encouraging some risk taking and reinforcing mentee involvement in initiatives.

6. Employee vision. The mentor introduces the mentee to considering new career training, clarifying skills, assessing options and resources, being confident with a prospective plan for career development, and being committed to accomplishing his or her goals.

Cohen reinforces the fact that this model should be seen as dynamic and fluid, not just as a theoretical framework of a mentor-mentee relationship. He describes some conditions that should be used for this model to be most effective:

- Planned sessions. In order for meaningful transactions between the mentor and mentee to occur, there must be adequate time on a scheduled basis for the mentor and mentee to meet.
- Holistic experience. The mentor and mentee need to interact over an extended time frame and must be free to talk about anything that influences the mentee's growth.
- Active participation. The mentor must participate in the mentee's activities and be involved in both personal and professional development. The mentor helps the mentee in transitions through significant life and work events.
- Ideal versus realistic perspective. The mentor should be able to function in all six dimensions of mentoring, but it is realistic that some mentors will be able to assume only some of the dimensions. In this case, multiple mentors will be highly useful.

Mentors should have an entrepreneurial side whereby they can encourage someone interested in doing something off the regular path to do so. The profession needs to empower nurses to use their creative ideas instead of giving them to the organization or physicians with whom they may have worked. What does "being an entrepreneur" mean? It can mean anything different that nurses do not usually do. Some say it is time for more nurse practitioners to open their own practice. Nurses can learn how to start up and operate a business. Independent contracting and consulting by nurse practitioners could be a good cash-flow business. If the operating costs were kept low enough to offer low-cost-visit charges, a primary care clinic could be very entrepreneurial in this day of high-premium insurance policies. People could pay cash and have insurance only for catastrophic events, so they would not be paying for high-cost insurance. Perhaps the insurance business would need to be overhauled to allow this. But this process does not appear far from reality. Whatever the entrepreneurial idea is, an effective mentor could assist the mentee in researching all angles. The decision to become an entrepreneur must be the mentee's, not forced on him or her by the mentor.

Every mentor mentors a little differently. This is fine because it is important to realize that one size does not fit all when it comes to mentoring. Effective mentoring is something we should all learn more about. Sometimes reading through an assessment such as those in *The Good Teacher Mentor: Setting the Standard for Support and Success* by Trubowitz and Robins (2003) is helpful. Fort (1995) offers a listing of 10 important mentoring rules that may also assist in improving the effectiveness of mentoring:

1. Almost anyone can be a mentor; in fact, undergraduates can mentor underclassmen.
2. Identify what you can offer a mentee.
3. Discuss how much guidance is going to be necessary and how much you are willing to offer. Determine how professional and personal you want to be.
4. Give criticism as well as reinforcement.
5. Invite mentees to informal social activities whenever possible so they can network.
6. Praise your mentees' talents to your colleagues.
7. Give new colleagues help in obtaining resources.
8. Be honest if a mentee is taking too much time or not enough with goal accomplishment.
9. Realize you cannot mentor everyone or be all that someone needs. Do not enable.
10. Mentors can be effective with mentees similar and different from themselves.

EXAMPLES OF EFFECTIVE AND INEFFECTIVE MENTORING

One study identified characteristics of mentees that mentors perceived to be most beneficial for a successful mentoring relationship (Allen, Poteet, & Russell, 2000). The mentee's potential as judged by the mentor and the mentee's need for help were identified as the top criteria. Another finding generated was that women mentors are most likely to choose a mentee based on the mentee's perceived ability than men mentors are. An example of effective mentoring follows:

> Cindy was a first-year master's of science in nursing student and just happened to go to a brown bag lunch with a friend who was majoring

in psychiatric nursing. The chair of this track was talking about her research in nursing care delivery and asked if anyone was interested in working with her on a research project. This faculty member had recently been funded to study specific patient variables on two separate units using different care modalities in a nearby hospital. Cindy volunteered and said she had experience as a staff nurse in the new care delivery mode. This was the beginning of a great mentorship that included both professional and personal development. The mentor guided Cindy through her thesis, two book chapters, and two journal articles, and she offered time to discuss other goals that Cindy had over the 2 years she was involved in her master's degree. Afterward the mentor wrote recommendations for her, included Cindy in another research project, helped Cindy obtain funding in her doctoral program, and served as a sounding board through doctoral study. Having had this excellent mentoring, Cindy was fortunate enough to know it was imperative to get involved with a similar type of mentor in her new job as a faculty member so she would be situated well for tenure and promotion.

An example of a need for mentoring follows:

Harry was a new nurse manager at a large health center and had received the mentoring that is considered needed for successful transformation from clinical level IV and charge nurse to nurse manager. He had actually been a charge or assistant nurse manager on two different units in the institution over the past 3 years. He never had the luxury of shadowing an experienced nurse manager. He also never had the opportunity to work on receiving or delivering constructive feedback with a mentor. He was well liked and considered by management as someone who had the correct leadership style and experience to make an effective nurse manager. After 6 months, he resigned and said the reason was that he just could not give negative feedback every day. He was able to identify the unit's challenges and was well received by the staff and attending physicians, but what he found impossible was being able to communicate directly to staff members when negative outcomes surfaced. Later he looked back and said he did not have the ability to word the feedback in a more positive fashion and so just blurted out what he felt and then felt so guilty that he ended up apologizing to the staff member.

Harry did not have the self-esteem to feel confident in his evaluations or the emotional intelligence to have the understanding that he had good working relationships with his staff and was expected to offer constructive criticism to the employees. He decided to become a nurse practitioner and chose a more solo versus team-oriented practice.

However, he soon realized he was experiencing a similar communication pattern with his patients who were not following his recommendations for a change in diet, alcohol, exercise, or smoking.

Could an effective mentoring experience have helped Harry? It is part of the mentor's job to assist the mentee in recognizing patterns of behavior that need modification. Through shadowing his mentor in managing conflicts and giving constructive criticism, Harry could have learned strategies to alter his communication techniques with employees needing feedback.

Unproductive mentorships can be dysfunctional for several reasons. Often, though, it is because mentors are too authoritative and critical or mentees have poor communication or no accountability. Whatever the reason, some guidelines to review might be helpful to identify an unproductive mentorship so it can be either stopped or corrected. Johnson and Huwe (2003) suggest that mentors and mentees ask the following questions if their relationship seems problematic:

- Are the needs of one or both the mentor and mentee no longer being met?
- Are the costs of the relationship outweighing the benefits for one of the partners?
- Is either member experiencing distress due to the relationship?

Johnson and Huwe (2003) identified the most frequent problems that occur in dysfunctional mentorships and offer the following characteristics of mentor-mentee dysfunction:

Poor match	Mismatch regarding communication style, work ethic, or clinical focus
Incompetent	Lack of mentor competence in clinical field and research areas
Emotional instability	Poor emotional intelligence and relationship skills
Neglect from mentor	Mentor function not evident; little time offered to mentee; no attention spent on mentee
Conflict	Focus is negative and accusatory, and no solutions are offered to correct problems
Violation of boundaries	Confusion; discomfort with relationship
Exploitation	Mentor manipulates mentee for his or her own good

Unethical behavior | Mentor encourages fraud or plagiarism
Abandonment by mentor | Mentor dies, is ill, has a job change, or abandons the mentee
Mentee dysfunction | Mentee procrastinates or is overly dependent on mentor

CHARACTERISTICS OF EFFECTIVE MENTORS

Most mentors want to be good mentors. They should first create and role-model a healthier lifestyle that decreases stress and balances career and family. Certainly this type of behavior may be a radical change for individuals who work in health care organizations that value a work schedule of 12-hour days. Perhaps it is time for leaders to make some big changes in the organizational culture in health care.

Sullivan (2004) suggests multiple strategies for best mentoring practices in chaotic organizations. A good mentor is a good leader, is credible, and commands respect. Mentors do not necessarily have to be in a position of authority, but they do have to have power and be politically astute. Being effective negotiators, excellent communicators, risk takers, change agents, creative thinkers, empowered, visionary, and culturally competent are all characteristics of a good leader that a mentor must have. Mentoring models refer to mentors as also being good teachers, facilitators, and advisers or coaches. The best mentors "bless" their students—that is, they call forth and affirm the mentee's life and career aspirations (Levinson et al., 1978).

Zachary (2000) offers the Mentoring Skills Inventory for mentors to assess their preparation to mentor. She recommends mentors acquire the following skills:

- Building and maintaining relationships
- Coaching
- Communicating
- Encouraging
- Facilitating
- Goal setting
- Guiding
- Managing conflict
- Problem solving
- Providing and receiving feedback
- Reflecting

Mentors can obtain practice in these areas by working with others who emulate these skills. Also, mentors who have had their own effective mentors can review experiences that they had with their mentor that involved these skills. Katzenbach (1996) talks about real change leaders (RCLs), who perhaps can be likened to nurses who are strong preceptors and mentors who seem to mentor everyone but tend not to be in the limelight. A three-year study by Katzenbach and associates demonstrates that the make-or-break factor for success in organizations that are undergoing extensive change is the frontline person, not the chief executive officer and senior executives. He identifies several of the common characteristics that RCLs portray:

- Consistently committed to the "better way"
- Courageous and diligent in challenging the standards and authority figures
- Dedicated in fighting for what they really believe in
- Empowering of self and others
- Sincerely caring about people and the organization
- Not out to be recognized and in the limelight
- Excellent sense of humor

There is little literature regarding mentoring women by women, but Fort (1995) cites that there is a mentoring gap for women. She believes it may be because women prefer to be mentored by women and there are fewer women in some disciplines who are at a point in their career to be a mentor. Also, many women believe they are not knowledgeable enough to be a mentor. She cites several myths about mentoring that may be helpful to review:

Myth: Having a mentor is the only way to succeed. *Fact:* Mentoring is a factor for success but is not essential for it.

Myth: Mentors should be older than mentees. *Fact:* Do not assume the older person should be the mentor in a relationship. Sometimes the more experienced person is younger.

Myth: A classic relationship is the best way to mentor. *Fact:* Networking and multiple mentoring models may be more helpful than some mentors.

Myth: Mentoring relationships must be long term to be truly useful. *Fact:* Significant mentoring can last over only a few days at a conference.

Myth: A person can have only one mentor at a time. *Fact:* Multiple mentoring through various networks may be extremely effective.

Myth: Mentoring is a one-way relationship, benefiting only the mentee. *Fact:* Mentors can gain large benefits from the mentee and the relationship.

Myth: Mentees must be invited by their mentors. *Fact:* Mentees should actively seek mentors.

Myth: When men mentor women, a sexual encounter is likely. *Fact:* Obviously this is not true but even with men mentoring men, there could be a sexual encounter.

Myth: Men are better mentors for women. *Fact:* Studies reveal that women mentors are more likely to affirm, encourage, and give examples rather than directions. Male mentors were found to direct mentees more and be disappointed if mentees did not follow their direction.

Myth: The mentor always knows best. *Fact:* No one person ever knows best.

Fort also offers some suggestions for all types of mentors in The (Woman) Mentor's 10 Commandments which are similar to Zachary's Mentoring Skills Inventory except for this one: a mentor cannot mentor everyone or be all that anyone needs. This sage advice echoes what is currently going on in nursing with the encouragement of using the multiple mentoring model. Mentors need to use their time wisely, and it appears that co-mentoring and multiple mentoring models may facilitate this. Kram (1983) reminds mentors that they need to teach the mentee the skills of the position and coach the mentee along the journey to gain confidence in order to be effective.

Hedgesen (1990) shares her findings about women who mentor and explores how their approaches differ from men's approaches to making decisions and priority setting. Based on her study of working with women leaders, she found that women are most interested in maintaining a more balanced life, that is, they want to be involved in their work and their family responsibilities. They view themselves as more than their image at work, and they see themselves at the center of things rather than at the top. Because of this, women create organizational structures that are not hierarchical. They see themselves as integrated in the whole system, which allows for more involvement with everyone in the organization. This information sheds light on how mentors should mentor women mentees.

BENEFITS OF BEING A MENTOR, PRECEPTOR, OR COACH

Starting with the fact that mentors can increase their own power from mentees' performance and loyalty (Restifo & Yoder, 2004), some mentors can receive credit for their recertification by precepting a graduate student

(Mobley, Gray, & Estep, 2003); bedside nurses can be promoted to the next clinical ladder by precepting; and a mentor can receive information for his or her own projects as well as grassroot rumors and talk from the organization through the mentee and his or her contacts (Mullen & Noe, 1999); there are countless benefits of mentoring. Gilley and Boughton (1996), Greggs-McQuilkin (2004), Ragins and Cotton (1999), and Kram (1985) add to the benefit list:

- Increased self-esteem
- Lifelong relationships in some cases
- Increased admiration by administration of your skills as mentor
- Increased leadership succession in the profession
- Psychological rewards of helping people
- Increased motivation and enthusiasm toward career
- Reinforcement that all of the work and sacrifice is worthwhile
- Generativity needs that can be complete

It is important to realize that mentors not only give but receive. McFarland et al. (1994) point out multiple ways for mentors to become part of an initiative or change that might have been originally developed for the mentee. Some nurse faculty have expertise in many facets of the faculty role and can greatly assist new faculty in obtaining tenure and promotion. However, many can learn new technology and be mentored by the junior faculty regarding grant funding or even become involved in new faculty's research initiatives and publications. Many of the newer faculty have been fortunate to have had mentoring in their doctoral programs and been introduced into networks that far exceed what faculty received who graduated 10 or more years ago from doctoral programs. It is hoped that the more experienced faculty will be empowered enough and have enough self-esteem to realize that reciprocal mentoring with new faculty will offer everyone benefits.

CONCLUSION

There are successful people who never had a mentor and nevertheless mentor many and accomplish great things. Many nurses receive more mentoring in a three-day conference span from collaborating and networking at the seminars than they do at their own institution. All mentors are not effective at mentoring, and some do not have helping the mentee as their purpose. Being a mentor should be an option, and not all senior people should be considered potential mentors. Rather, these senior people can contribute to the organization in other ways.

It is more important to foster a mentoring culture in nursing so that more nurses can get connected to each other and to individuals in other disciplines. Partnering with other agencies, collaborating whenever possible, and reciprocal mentoring are what the profession needs in order to advance itself. This chapter has suggested many strategies to provide best mentoring practice.

Bolman and Deal (2001) provide a story of one man's search for soul and spirit using a mentor. The authors define *soul* as "personal and unique, grounded in depths of personal experience" (p. 9). They describe *spirit* as "transcendent and all embracing, it is the universal source, the oneness of all things" (p. 9). Their book is a powerful one for mentors to review because they explain how we all need to relearn how to lead with soul and spirit, and that soul, spirit, and faith belong at the heart of leadership. Nursing needs to have more mentoring for bedside nurses and for the members of professional organizations in order to foster a mentoring culture. Today there are mentoring relationships available for many advanced practice nurses, nurses in administration, nurses involved in leading the professional organizations, junior faculty, and doctoral students.

REFERENCES

Allen, T., Poteet, M., & Russell, J. (2000). Protégé selection by mentors: What makes the difference? *Journal of Organizational Behavior, 21,* 271–283.

Andrews, M., & Wallis, M. (1999). Mentorship in nursing: A literature review. *Journal of Advanced Nursing, 29,* 201–207.

Bell, C. (2002). *Managers as mentors: Building partnerships for learning.* San Francisco: Berrett-Koehler.

Block, P. (1996). *Stewardship: Choosing service over self-interest.* San Francisco: Berrett-Koehler.

Bolman, L., & Deal, T. (2001). *Leading with soul: An uncommon journey of spirit.* San Francisco: Jossey-Bass.

Cohen, N. (1999). *The manager's pocket guide to effective mentoring.* Amherst, MA: HRD.

Fort, D. (Ed.). (1995). *A hand up: Women mentoring women in science.* Washington, DC: Association for Women in Science.

Gilley, J., & Boughton, N. (1996). *Stop managing, start coaching.* Chicago: Irwin.

Greggs-McQuilkin, D. (2004). Mentoring really matters: Motivate and mentor a colleague. *MEDSURG Nursing, 13,* 209–210.

Hedgesen, S. (1990). *The female advantage: Women's ways of leadership*. New York: Doubleday Currency.

Johnson, W., & Huwe, J. (2003). *Getting mentored: In graduate school*. Washington, DC: American Psychological Association.

Katzenbach, J. (1996). *Real change leaders: How you can create growth and high performance at your company*. New York: Three Rivers Press.

Kouzes, J., & Posner, B. (1993). *Credibility: How leaders gain and lose it, why people demand it*. San Francisco: Jossey-Bass.

Kram, K. (1983). Phases of the mentor relationship. *Academy of Management Journal, 26*, 608–625.

Lanser, E. (2000). Reaping the benefits of mentorship. *Healthcare Executive, 15*, 18–23.

Levinson, D., Darrow, C., Klein, E., Levinson, M., & McKee, B. (1978). *The seasons of a man's life*. New York: Knopf.

Lowney, C. (2003). *Heroic leadership: Best practices from a 450-year old company that changed the world*. Chicago: Loyola Press.

Luna, G., & Cullen, D. (1996). *Empowering the faculty: Mentoring redirected and renewed*. Washington, DC: George Washington University Press.

McCall, M. (1998). *High flyers: Developing the next generation of leaders*. Boston: Harvard Business School Press.

McFarland, L., Senn, L., & Childress, J. (1994). *21st century leadership: Dialogues with 100 top leaders*. New York: Leadership Press.

Mobley, C., Gray, B., & Estep, S. (2003). "Growing" nurse practitioners: Mentoring strategies for preceptors. *Advance for Nurse Practitioners, 3*, 51–54.

Mullen, E., & Noe, R. (1999). The mentoring information exchange: When do mentors seek information from their protégés? *Journal of Organizational Behavior, 20*, 233–333.

Myrick, F. (2002). Preceptorship and critical thinking in nursing education. *Journal of Nursing Education, 41*,154–164.

Ragins, B., & Cotton, J. (1999). Mentor functions and outcomes: A comparison of men and women in formal and informal mentoring relationships. *Journal of Applied Psychology, 84*, 529–550.

Reardon, K. (2004). *The skilled negotiator: Mastering the language of engagement*. San Francisco: Jossey-Bass.

Restifo, V., & Yoder, L. (2004). Partnership: Making the most of mentoring. *Nursing Spectrum, 8*, 16–19.

Robinson-Walker, C. (1999). *Women and leadership in health care: The journey to authenticity and power*. San Francisco: Jossey-Bass.

Ross, A., Wenzel, F., & Mitlyng, J. (2002). *Leadership for the future: Core competencies in health care*. Chicago: Health Administration Press.

Shea, G. (1999). *Making the most of being mentored*. Menlo Park, CA: Crisp Learning.

Sinetar, M. (1998). *The mentor's spirit: Life lessons on leadership and the art of encouragement*. New York: St. Martin's Press.

Stone, F. (1999). *Coaching, counseling, and mentoring: How to choose and use the right technique to boost employee performance.* New York: American Management Association.

Sullivan, C. (2004). *How to mentor in the midst of change* (2nd ed.). Alexandria, VA: Association for Supervision and Curriculum Development.

Trubowitz, S., & Robins, M. (2003). *The good teacher mentor: Setting the standard for support and success.* New York: Teachers College Press.

Watkins, M., & Bazerman, M. (2003). Predictable surprises: The disasters you should have seen coming. *Harvard Business Review, 81,* 72–80.

Werner, J. (2002). Mentoring and its potential nursing role. *Creative Nursing Journal, 3,* 13–14.

Zachary, L. (2000). *The mentor's guide: Facilitating effective learning relationships.* San Francisco: Jossey-Bass.

Zey, M. (1990). *The mentor connection: Strategic alliances in corporate life.* New Brunswick, NJ: Transaction.

CHAPTER 6

The Mentee Perspective on How Best to Become Empowered

The explosion of knowledge today is so tremendous that it is impossible for one nurse to know all there is to know about a topic in nursing; rather, nurses need to work collaboratively to be able to provide best practice. This is also true of mentors: no one mentor can provide everything a mentee needs. Today, nurses need to work within a mentoring culture with more than one mentor to accomplish their goals and become self-empowered. These goals will not only be those of the mentees and the mentors, but will also reflect the goals of the organization and advancement of the profession.

Most would agree that the majority of people do not succeed strictly on their own and without help from anyone. But there are people who say they have never been mentored and think they have reached the pinnacle of success solely on their own. It is important for nurses to review their careers and acknowledge those who have contributed to their career. Although many have not had the classic mentoring that some nurses may have wished to have experienced, it is most likely today that faculty, researchers, and administrators have had some mentoring. By realizing the impact that various individuals have had on one's career, and maybe even one's personal life, it seems that more nurses might extend themselves to encourage other nurses or even offer to mentor someone. Being able to recognize others' influence indicates confidence in one's expertise and knowledge, and high self-esteem. It is a sign of being empowered to be able to credit others. Many (Daloz, 1999; Murray, 2001; Parks, 2000; Shea, 1999; Sinetar, 1998) say those who have been mentored will most likely mentor others. Therefore, a pool of potential mentors, coaches, and preceptors is available to nurse mentees. It is important for mentees to look for mentors, preceptors, role models, and coaches in order to foster more of a mentoring culture in nursing. This chapter describes effective mentee relationships, ideas for choosing an effective mentor, suggestions for maximizing the potential for being chosen by an effective mentor, and the benefits and possible negatives of being in a mentoring relationship.

EFFECTIVE RELATIONSHIP FOR THE MENTEE

Chapters 4 and 5 explored how to set up and develop a mentorship and the characteristics that describe an effective mentor (Table 4.1) and an effective mentee (Table 4.2), and how to maintain a successful mentorship or preceptorship. Much of this influences the effectiveness of the relationship on the mentee as well.

Mentees should have interpersonal maturity, self-confidence, experience in managing stress, ability to benefit from constructive feedback, and personal determination. Shea (1999), Luna and Cullen (1996), and Schweibert (2000) describe findings from their research that include identification of characteristics of effective mentees:

- Emotional stability. The person has a good sense of awareness of who he or she is. Others perceive the individual as self-confident and having a balanced life.
- High sense of locus of control. The individual is committed to making a difference and has a sense his or her work will influence events.
- Interest in learning. The mentee is willing to learn from others and receive feedback on his or her work without being defensive.
- Emotional intelligence. The person can develop relationships easily with others.
- Achievement focused. The individual has hardiness, that is, a strong work ethic, and follows through with work.

Nurse educators need to foster these characteristics in students so that more nurses can benefit from being involved in the mentoring culture, participating in a network, partnering with others to share resources and talents, and being prepared to mentor others. Of course, there are always arrogant people who think they need no mentoring and also those who receive expert mentoring but still cannot deliver any outcomes from the relationship. Is it the mentor's fault that the mentee did not accomplish his or her goals? Probably not. In most instances, it is the environment or the mentee's not accepting accountability for his or her commitments that mitigates a successful mentorship. It does seem that the most successful outcomes of mentorships are related to mentees' possessing characteristics previously listed that can be acquired by working with a mentor-leader and developing one's own leadership skills. A student nurse who began to acquire these skills would have an accelerated growth process as a new graduate nurse.

Suen and Chow (2001) described the perceptions of undergraduate nursing students regarding the effectiveness of their mentors—actually, preceptors. The findings demonstrate that students felt their preceptor treated them like guests on their units and did not welcome them as team members. This was considered absence of the befriending role. Also, students felt that the mentor did not fulfill the adviser role in most instances. However, they felt that the other three roles of assistant, counselor, and guide were well fulfilled. So since the study is about preceptors, not classic mentors, the researchers understood why the friendship and career advisement functions were perceived as absent. The results of this study reaffirm the importance of mentors and mentees or preceptors and preceptees being told exactly what to expect prior to a preceptorship or mentorship. It also validates the need to differentiate between the classic mentor role and all of the other roles that are often referred to as *mentor*.

An important skill that mentees need to embrace is uncertainty and to be able to respond flexibly in situations. New nurses need to have the ability to work in uncertain circumstances and make decisions as the time evolves. They have to have a skeleton plan that is focusing their day's work, but they also have to realize that anything can happen so they need to be able to adjust readily. This correlates well to Benner's research that resulted in the Acquisition of Skill Model. The less experienced nurse tends to be more task oriented and rigid, as well as more focused on the parts of a patient and not necessarily the whole patient. As novices gain more experience, it becomes easier for them to see more globally—that is, they can begin to see the whole patient. By observing more experienced nurses practice flexibility, manage uncertainty, and favorably react to change, mentees can gain confidence to practice these skills themselves.

Clampitt and DeKoch (2001) provide evidence that it is more efficient and rewarding to embrace uncertainty than try to eliminate it. They describe that leaders know they can never know everything and that not knowing is quite legitimate. More of this type of thinking needs to be fostered so the morale of the organization will stay high and creative strategies to embrace change will occur. These authors developed the Working Climate Survey, which measures one's tendency to embrace uncertainty and provides insight into one's comfort with uncertainty and ambiguity. Clampitt and DeKoch recommend that mentees take the Working Climate

Survey to understand how they view uncertainty. Their book, *Embracing Uncertainty: The Essence of Leadership*, presents this tool with interpretive guidelines and offers suggestions to being able to be less controlling and more flexible in meeting challenges.

A significant quality that mentors can help mentees do for themselves is empowering them to cut loose from their own imposed limits so they can maximize their ability to grow (Jaworski, 1998). Often it is these self-imposed barriers that curtail growth for individuals. By offering opportunities for nurses and students to shadow a nurse leader, they can learn how to take risks, manage conflict, negotiate for what is important to one's unit or position on an issue, and countless other skills that will empower them to succeed in their career. McLane (2005) presents a narrative on a day in the life of a manager that is helpful to students and nurses beginning their first clinical day on a unit. Shadowing a staff nurse gives them an opportunity to observe a staff nurse as well as to see how a unit operates prior to accepting a position on a unit. It would behoove every individual to take advantage of such an observational experience. There are two resources that mentees can review to determine if they are ready for a mentorship: a list of do's and don'ts for mentees in *The Good Teacher Mentor: Setting the Standard for Support and Success* by Trubowitz and Robins (2003) and the protégé self-assessment by Johnson and Huwe (2003). Both inventories are composed of questions regarding their perceptions of their own communication, work ethic, self-esteem, ability to receive feedback, goals for their future, and needs from a mentorship.

The profession of nursing benefits if each doctoral student has an opportunity to work in a classic mentoring relationship. Byrne and Keefe (2002) describe their experience working together with a National Institutes of Health grant in maternal-infant research. They analyzed personal reflections over the four-year working period and concluded that the mentee primary investigator must be organized, focused, and have self-direction. They also found the mentor primary investigator must have generativity, altruism, and expertise to have a successful experience.

Wills and Kaiser (2002) describe several strategies (know what you want, be realistic with your expectations, network with everyone you can, negotiate for opportunities, and evaluate your learning as you go) for assisting junior faculty mentees to be the most productive in maximizing their scholarly productivity with their mentors. The same types of strategies will assist doctoral students to be successful within the mentoring culture. Montgomery (2001) describes that a good match between a mentor and mentee includes a supportive mentor who is trustworthy; having established, clear boundaries regarding responsibilities; sharing consistent personal philosophies and similar work habits; and having good communication skills. Her mentoring experience as a doctoral student in an academic setting with a head of the nursing division for one and one-half days each week for nine months is a good example of what mentoring should be. She described her experience as including working alongside the mentor to accomplish the work of leading the undergraduate program and engaging in administrative learning experiences throughout the university.

Multiple leaders (Miller, 2003; Schwiebert, 2000; Sullivan, 2004; Zachary, 2000) point out the benefits of mentoring regarding increased self-confidence with various skills and evolving increased self-esteem. They say being a mentee promotes self-development, which in turn has multiple positive influences on one's career trajectory as well as patient care. Dossey, Selanders, Beck, and Attewell (2005) share ideas on reaching for goals and following their visions in order to make a difference. They say nurses can influence the care of patients in an enormous way. *Ever yours: Florence Nightingale: Selected letters* is a collection of Nightingale's annual letters that she wrote to nurses a century ago. It also includes the infamous essay written in 1893, "Sick-Nursing and Health-Nursing," which, even one century ago, was citing the importance of nurses promoting health to prevent sickness.

Many nurses do not find a mentor unless they go to graduate school, become a midlevel manager, or are in some expanded role. It is nevertheless advantageous for every nurse to find a mentor who can offer leadership skills through coaching, role modeling, or precepting (Restifo & Yoder, 2004). The most likely way a staff nurse will become part of the mentoring culture is if he or she began as a student. Educators in associate and baccalaureate programs need to be involved in assisting students to make more mentoring connections. These students will benefit from preceptors and coaches who advise and role-model them along the way to becoming a graduate nurse. Faculty must be part of the mentoring culture for these students. However, students must also go outside the college and look for other mentoring connections. There is a greater tendency today for faculty to get involved with graduate students rather than with undergraduates. This is due to the benefits faculty perceive they can receive from graduate students, such as assistance with their research or connections with a graduate's work setting. These types of reciprocal mentoring outcomes offer a more direct payback when it comes to career advancement and promotion. All new clinical staff have a preceptor in their first few weeks, but generally after completion of the orientation program, there is no further relationship. There may be communication between the newly hired staff and more experienced staff member if the new staff member initiates contact. So how can the mentee or preceptee forge ahead to keep or develop a support system? By encouraging the communication between one's faculty and preceptor, the mentee will develop a mentoring matrix. This matrix will gradually begin to evolve and bring in more connections. It takes time, thought, and some work for mentees to encourage their mentors to keep communication flowing. A mentee who recognizes the mentor's contributions during the relationship with kind words, a thank-you card, e-mail or telephone call, or giving a small token of thanks will motivate the mentors to keep connected. These connections are paramount for the overall development of a mentoring culture in nursing.

CHOOSING A MENTOR OR, MORE APPROPRIATELY, MENTORS

Wolf (2002) and Shea (1999) recommend that mentees try to learn multiple viewpoints from several people; learn all that is possible about an organization; network with others; practice skills with experienced people; and keep a record of the mentoring experiences. Shea (1999) says mentees can make the most of their relationship by following some simple rules: articulate goals clearly with the mentor, become comfortable with the mentor, establish trust with the mentor, and be willing to be flexible. Shea further suggests that mentees be aware that mentors are looking for mentees interested in a formal mentoring program who are

- self-empowered;
- not living in an extreme stressful environment;
- practiced in conflict management;
- ethical;
- interested in improving communication skills;
- caring;
- practiced in team building;
- expert in an area of content that has potential for funding;
- trustworthy;
- assertive.

Grossman (2005) conducted focus groups with senior nursing students who had experienced a semester of shadowing a leader in health care. The students identified the following as characteristics for prospective mentors to possess:

- Commitment
- Willing to give frequent constructive feedback
- Collaborates with mentee to revise goals as mentorship evolves
- Perceives mentee's input as valuable
- Demonstrates respect for mentee in the organization
- Able to empower others and assist one to empower self
- Provides experiences so student is shadowing and not doing delegated assignments
- Demonstrates creative and effective problem solving and lets the mentee observe
- Demonstrates effective communication skills and lets the mentee observe
- Advocates for change and flexibility
- Shares hints on balancing professional and personal life

Knowing what to look for in a potential mentor is helpful. Oermann (2002) stresses the importance for new graduates to be open to listening and taking advice from experienced nurses in order to manage the challenges of working in the hospital. She recommends that mentees go out and find a mentor since mentors do not necessarily come to potential mentees. Oermann reinforces that finding a person to be a mentor will most likely not be the preceptor who was assigned during the new graduate's orientation. In addition, most individuals will need to seek out more long-term mentoring during their careers rather than think they will establish a mentor-mentee relationship during their educational program. Parks (2000) reminds us that mentoring communities are new forms of support that are developing for young adults. Nurses can take advantage of this philosophy by networking with people outside health care as well. It seems that the person desiring mentoring needs to seek out people in their lives to be part of a network of encouragement for them. The 20- and 30-year-olds need to find time to network with their peers and families for support and encouragement.

BENEFITS AND POSSIBLE NEGATIVES
OF BEING A MENTEE

Kanter (1977) feels mentees will benefit from a mentor with professional power by acquiring reflective power. This is evident in graduate education and should become more and more obvious as junior nursing faculty become federally funded due to their mentoring connections. It is crucial for nurses proceeding to academia to have powerful mentors who can assist them with this necessary component for success as a faculty member. So too, powerful mentors will assist nurse administrators to climb the ladder and obtain the coveted nurse executive positions in health care agencies. It would be beneficial for all aspiring to higher positions to read Kanter's book, *Men and Women of the Corporation* (1977).

Mentoring theory proposes that relationships change over time (Chao, 1997; Kram, 1983, 1985). Kram's stages of the classic mentoring relationship can teach mentees what to anticipate, so they will be better prepared to maximize the benefits they can achieve from the relationship. There are four stages:

1. Initiation. The mentor and mentee have their first interaction with each other and try to emotionally connect. There is uncertainty during this first stage, so it is crucial for them to identify similarities and use these to connect. If the dyad can get over differences in this phase, they can proceed to a positive relationship.
2. Cultivation. A tremendous amount of career and psychosocial mentoring can occur during this stage. By attempting to shift toward a mutual exchange of resources and learning, the mentee will benefit the mentor. This in turn will motivate the mentor to make more connections for the mentee. When one of the dyad feels a need for change, this stage will end.
3. Separation. This is generally spontaneous and occurs when the mentee has increased autonomy. Some will stop all contacts, and others will proceed to stage 4.
4. Redefinition. This stage allows for whatever the mentor and mentee want. The mentee can gain the most by maintaining a collegial relationship with the mentor, or perhaps they have become friends.

Restifo and Yoder (2004) describe some of the common benefits of being mentored: obtaining advice for career advancement, learning new knowledge, gaining awareness of organizational culture, and learning multiple skills such as stress management, writing, teaching, and statistical analysis methods. Also, mentees gain a solid sense of ethics, networking opportunities, organizational savvy, and improved employability. There are multiple positive outcomes that are a product of effective mentoring relationships. Benefits for students who receive mentoring and precepting have been described. Perhaps the biggest benefits perceived by students, faculty, and preceptors have been increased confidence in performing skills, time management, and improved ability to make independent decisions (McGregor, 1999).

Eisen (2001), Glass and Walter (2000), Broscious and Saunders (2001), and Waddell and Dunn (2005) discuss the advantages of being involved in peer mentoring networks. Both give good examples of how peer coaching assists with the transfer of knowledge to clinical practice. They point out the benefits of being involved in a voluntary, nonevaluative, and mutually beneficial relationship.

There are negative aspects to having a mentorship. This section refers to the classic mentoring relationship and not preceptorships. Eby, Butts, Lockwood, and Simon (2004) found that negative mentoring can be powerful in predicting a mentee's negative outcomes over and above positive mentoring. In fact, it is better to have no mentor than to have a negative one. Social exchange theory says that some relationships involve positive and negative experiences, whereas some are just positive or just negative or even fail to meet one's needs and are neutral but not damaging.

There is little research on negative mentoring, but one of the biggest negatives that mentees have experienced is mentors who take credit for the mentee's work. It is possible to have both a positive and negative mentor behavior from one mentor. The mentee will have to assess if working with the mentor to receive the positive benefits outweighs the negative ones. Some negative outcomes of a bad mentorship include a lack of networking with others; being associated with a mentor without integrity, which may cause others to view the mentee similarly; receiving little to no coaching or feedback; and having no exposure to the organization or profession. Realization of being involved in a bad relationship is the first step. Then the mentee needs to consult with peers to validate if his or her suspicions about what is happening with the mentor are accurate. If the mentee is involved with a faculty person, it may be difficult to terminate the mentorship; however, the mentee should seek advice from the faculty's chair or dean. Findings from research (N = 84 mentees) by Eby et al. (2004) warn mentees to be aware of potential negative mentoring experiences—for example:

- Mismatch of mentor and mentee regarding values, work styles, and personality—the most frequently reported problem
- Mentors who neglect or intentionally exclude mentees from important meetings; these mentors are perceived as self-absorbed
- Manipulative behavior by the mentor, as when the mentor takes credit for the mentee's work or deliberately sabotages the mentee
- Mentors with poor communication skills
- Mentors with no specific nursing knowledge, clinical expertise, or research skills

- Mentors who have a negative attitude toward their work, the organization, or the mentee, or have personal problems

It is wise to go into a mentor relationship knowing what each expects to receive from the mentorship. Setting up a contract seems to be going too far; however, it may be important to avoid some of the pitfalls of negative mentorships. One would hope that only a few such relationships actually turn out negative. This optimism would put the odds in the mentee's favor that someone who is in the position to mentor others is reputable enough not to have negative motives. Mentees need to be proactive and assess if there are any negative motives (the mentor needs to be dominant, or has unwanted work to delegate, or needs to exert power, for example). Perhaps it would be more helpful to determine what the mentor's track record is with mentoring and communicate with previous mentees regarding their experience. It would seem prudent for mentees not to go into a mentorship blindly since it is a considerable commitment for doctoral students, as well as junior faculty. There is little research that identifies variables to successfully match mentors and mentees. Shea (1999) warns mentees not to make assumptions about expectations from the relationship that are incorrect. He has found that unsuccessful matches occur more often if there are cultural differences between the mentor and mentee.

CONCLUSION

Nurses need to be passionate about their work. How better to be motivated than by observing colleagues who are excited and successful with their aspirations? Everyone can remember a colleague who was the best and at the top of his or her career but never moved on to conquer more mountains. For some reason, they felt stuck. Others who were movers and shakers grew tired of the status quo work setting and joined more ambitious institutions. As some work environments get more toxic, employees lose their self-esteem and self-empowerment, and become one of the losers. Donald Trump says on his television show *The Apprentice* that he has learned over and over that "one who works with losers will eventually become a loser." This seems to be true. Mentees who belong to mentoring connections will be less likely to fall into a loser environment, and they will have the support and strength of their mentoring network to pull themselves out. Mentees need to realize they are not entitled to be a winner but have to work hard to achieve success. They have to take risks, try new things, and accept change (Porter-O'Grady, 1997). Mentees need to be involved in peer and multiple mentoring networks. By improving their leadership skills through mentoring, mentees will be able to help themselves as well as the profession. Parks (2000) recommends that it is more important than ever before to assist the new generation in pursuing their dreams rather than focusing on self-interest. Mentors need to role-model well today in order to influence the future professional nurses.

REFERENCES

Broscious, S., & Saunders, D. (2001). Peer coaching. *Nurse Educator, 26,* 212–214.

Byrne, M., & Keefe, M. (2002). Building research competence in nursing through mentoring. *Journal of Nursing Scholarship, 34,* 391–396.

Chao, G. (1997). Mentoring phases and outcomes. *Journal of Vocational Behavior, 51,* 15–28.

Clampitt, P., & DeKoch, R. (2001). *Embracing uncertainty: The essence of leadership.* Armonk, NY: M. E. Sharpe.

Daloz, L. (1999). *Mentor: Guiding the journey of adult learners* (2nd ed.). San Francisco: Jossey-Bass.

Dossey, B., Selanders, L., Beck, D. M., & Attewell, A. (2005). *Florence Nightingale today: Healing leadership global action.* Washington, DC: American Nurses Association.

Eby, L., Butts, M., Lockwood, A., & Simon, S. (2004). Protégés' negative mentoring experiences: Construct development and nomological validation. *Personnel Psychology, 57,* 411–448.

Eisen, M. (2001). Peer based professional development viewed through the lens of transformative learning. *Holistic Nursing Practice, 16,* 30–42.

Glass, N., & Walter, R. (2000). An experience of peer mentoring with student nurses: Enhancement of personal and professional growth. *Journal of Nursing Education, 39,* 155–160.

Grossman, S. (2005). Developing leadership through shadowing a leader in health care. In H. Feldman & M. Greenberg (Eds.), *Educating for leadership* (pp. 266–278). New York: Springer Publishing.

Jaworski, J. (1998). *Synchronicity: The inner path of leadership.* San Francisco: Berrett-Koehler.

Johnson, W., & Huwe, J. (2003). *Getting mentored: In graduate school.* Washington, DC: American Psychological Association.

Kanter, R. (1977). *Men and women of the corporation.* New York: Basic Books.

Kram, K. (1983). Phases of the mentor relationship. *Academy of Management Journal, 26,* 608–625.

Kram, K. (1985). Mentoring in the workplace. In D. Hall (Ed.), *Career development in organizations* (pp. 160–201). San Francisco: Jossey-Bass.

Luna, G., & Cullen, D. (1996). *Empowering the faculty: Mentoring redirected and renewed.* Washington, DC: George Washington University Press.

McGregor, R. (1999). A precepted experience for senior nursing students. *Nurse Educator, 24*, 13–16.

McLane, S. (2005). A day in the life of a manager: Incorporating leadership, management, and role modeling. *Oncology Nursing Forum, 32*, 23–25.

Miller, T. (2003). *Building and managing a career in nursing.* Indianapolis: Sigma Theta Tau International.

Montgomery, K. (2001). Administrative substance: A mentoring experience. *Nursing Leadership Forum, 6*, 17–20.

Murray, M. (2001). *Beyond the myths and magic of mentoring: How to facilitate an effective mentoring process* (2nd ed.). San Francisco: Jossey-Bass.

Oermann, M. (2002). Stresses and challenges for new graduates in hospitals. *Nurse Education Today, 22*, 225–230.

Parks, S. D. (2000). *Big questions, worthy dreams: Mentoring young adults in their search for meaning, purpose, and faith.* San Francisco: Jossey-Bass.

Porter-O'Grady, T. (1997). The private practice of nursing: The gift of entrepreneurialism. *Nursing Administration Quarterly, 22*, 32–29.

Restifo, V., & Yoder, L. (2004). Partnership: Making the most of mentoring. *Nursing Spectrum, 8*, 15–19.

Robinson-Walker, C. (1999). *Women and leadership in health care: The journey to authenticity and power.* San Francisco: Jossey-Bass.

Schwiebert, V. (2000). *Mentoring: Creating connected, empowered relationships.* Alexandria, VA: American Counseling Association.

Shea, G. (1999). *Making the most of being mentored: How to grow from a mentoring partnership.* Menlo Park, CA: Crisp Publications.

Sinetar, M. (1998). *The mentor's spirit: Life lessons on leadership and the art of encouragement.* New York: St. Martin's Press.

Suen, L., & Chow, F. (2001). Students' perceptions of the effectiveness of the effectiveness of mentors in an undergraduate nursing programme in Hong Kong. *Journal of Advanced Nursing, 36*, 505–511.

Sullivan, C. (2004). *How to mentor in the midst of change* (2nd ed.). New York: Association for Supervision and Curriculum Development.

Trubowitz, S., & Robins, M. (2003). *The good teacher mentor: Setting the standard for support and success.* New York: Teachers College Press.

Vicinus, M., & Nergaard, B. (1990). *Ever yours: Florence Nightingale: Selected letters.* Boston: Harvard University Press.

Waddell, D., & Dunn, N. (2005). Peer coaching: The next step in staff development. *Journal of Continuing Education in Nursing, 36*, 84–89.

Wills, C., & Kaiser, L. (2002). Navigating the course of scholarly productivity: The protégé's role in mentoring. *Nursing Outlook 50*, 61–66.

Wolf, G. (2002). What the books don't tell you: Personal mentoring from one of the nation's leading health care administrators. *Journal of Clinical Systems Management, 4*, 7.

Zachary, L. (2002). *The mentor's guide.* San Francisco: Jossey-Bass.

CHAPTER 7

Mentoring Generates
Outcome Measurements

There is a lack of documented results of the effects of mentoring. Most relationships and programs are evaluated with qualitative open-ended questions regarding mentor and mentee perceptions of the experience. Commonly thought expected results of mentoring are that mentees will be able to accomplish goals more quickly having had a mentor than if they did not and staffing needs will be more adequately met. The ultimate outcome of mentoring is for mentees to become professionally socialized (Bandura, 1977). Precepting programs and other university-hospital partnerships generally measure their success by the number of nurses recruited and retained by the health care agency sponsoring the preceptorship. Student preceptorships and shadowing programs are measured by collecting student perceptions of their experiences, preceptors' perceptions of student performance, and possibly student critical thinking scores or some other tangible outcome that is evaluated before and after the preceptorship. There is a need for outcome studies regarding mentoring that measure mentee critical thinking, clinical decision making, leadership development, and possibly a correlation to progression on Benner's novice to expert continuum. There is an enormous need for more outcome measurement to document the efficacy of all mentoring programs. This chapter presents outcome implications related to mentoring for the profession, the organization, patient consumers, mentors, and mentees.

THE PROFESSION

It would be helpful to assess the variables that affect a nurse's ability to be a successful mentor. One would assume these variables would come from the definition of mentoring and include the length of the mentoring relationship the mentor is involved in, whether the mentorship was informal or formally assigned, and the organizational culture in which the mentor and mentee worked. No studies of how these variables influence mentoring were found. Another variable, mentoring potential, was cited by Fields (1991) to be identified by 125 recruited mentors as a significant predictor of a good mentoring relationship. This finding is corroborated by Shea (1999), Daloz (1999), Kram (1983), and Roberts (2000). Literature supports that mentoring is viewed as an important developmental process fostering professional maturation, career satisfaction, and the growth of strong, competent leaders in nursing (Stewart & Krueger, 1996; Anthony et al., 2005; Shea, 1999) says the closeness and cooperation that develops between a mentor and mentee over time is what produces great energy and creativity. It is this great outpouring of ideas that assists the mentee and mentor to accomplish such success. Think of some of the great mentor-mentee pairs: Socrates and Plato, Haydn and Beethoven, and Freud and Jung. It is the drawing out of the potential from the mentee and even perhaps from the mentor that makes a huge difference

Fields (1991) cites research indicating the majority of nurse leaders have or have had mentors and offers accounts of how their mentor relationships cultivated their abilities and assisted in providing opportunities for these mentee-leaders. The importance of mentor's introducing mentees to influential people who can help their careers may be the most significant outcome for the profession. By creating a mentoring culture, the profession can accomplish much more than if individual nurses work in isolation.

Mentoring is positively correlated with salary growth, career progression, increased self-esteem, job and career satisfaction, and decreased turnover intentions for the mentee (Goran, 2001). All of these outcomes positively influence the profession by improving the image of nursing. Bower (2000) describes another important outcome of mentoring as the relationships that are generated. These tend to result in lasting and unique colleague contacts. Gilligan (1993) agrees that a mentorship is a professional friendship and reinforces the concept of developing a mentoring culture throughout the profession. Gilligan studied the career development of nurses and found that mentoring relationships enhanced skill building and increased self-confidence in the mentees. Influential nurse leaders recognized the significant assistance that they received from their mentors and feel they extended this influence to others. In Gilligan's study of nationally recognized nurse influentials (N = 71), approximately 83% reported having had at least one successful mentorship, and 93% of the mentees reported mentoring others as their career progressed. Gilligan promotes the idea that developing visionary leadership through mentoring is an obligation for nurse leaders. Research cites that effective mentoring positively influences mentee leadership skills (Murray et al., 1998; Trossman, 1998). This has a significant impact on the profession.

Aiken's (2005; Aiken, Havens, & Sloan, 2000) studies of professional practice at magnet hospitals are being linked with Kanter's (1979) investigation of workplace empowerment and demonstrate that magnet hospitals allow for more nurse empowerment (Laschinger, Almost, & Tuer-Hodes, 2003). This outcome is directly related to mentoring and effective leadership by nurses who practice in magnet hospitals. But Kramer and Schmalenberg (2003) report in their study of staff nurse perceptions of autonomy that 26% of magnet hospital nurses reported situations of unsupported or even no autonomy. So it is not feasible to make sweeping generalizations that all nurses who work at magnet hospitals perceive themselves as empowered or that they have received effective mentoring.

The American Association of Critical Care Nurses (AACN) has recently released *The AACN Standards for Establishing and Sustaining Healthy Work Environments: A Journey to Excellence* (2005b). This document focuses on six areas that are mandatory if a safe and healthy work environment is to exist in hospitals: communication, collaboration, decision making, staffing, recognition, and leadership. The leaders need to come forward from the profession and take on responsibility for maintaining these standards. Nurses can and are stepping up to the plate in many settings and with more coaching and mentoring will join the crusade to establish a mentoring culture that will help produce a healthy work environment. More and more it is the nurse manager and other nurse leaders who need to bridge the hospital executives and bedside nurses so that organizational and professional goals can be achieved. With the current demand for nurses, it is imperative that nurse leaders create positive work environments, socialize nurses to adapt new ways for delivering nursing care, and allow for development of leadership skills by all. Laschinger, Wong, and McMahon (1999) found that staff nurses feel empowered when their leaders identify meaning in their work, increase staff involvement with decision making, and offer a positive work environment. Feeling empowered will provide the momentum for nurses to want to stay in their positions and recruit more nurses.

ORGANIZATION AND PATIENT CONSUMERS

Clinton (2002) cites that magnet hospitals retain nurses an average of twice as long as nonmagnet institutions and have proven their ability to attract and keep nurses. Aiken et al. (2000) called magnet hospitals "nursing's best kept secret" and demonstrate that work environments in these hospitals have higher nurse satisfaction and improved patient outcomes.

The magnet hospital movement began in 1980 and resulted in a book, *Forces of Magnetism*, which was revised and is currently entitled, *Magnet Hospitals Revisited* (McClure & Hinshaw, 2002). The program is based on the American Nurses Association's *Scope and Standards for Nurse Administrators* (2004). Magnet recognition is a process that assesses the implementation of 14 evidence-based standards of nursing excellence (American Nurses Credentialing Center, 2003):

1. Assessment
2. Diagnosis
3. Identification of outcomes
4. Planning
5. Implementation
6. Evaluation
7. Quality of care and administrative practice
8. Performance appraisal
9. Education
10. Collegiality
11. Ethics
12. Collaboration
13. Research
14. Resource utilization

Agencies can apply for magnet status every 4 years. (For more information regarding this program, log on to www.nursingworld.org/ancc/magnet.html.) Aiken (2005) describes results of a study that paired four magnet hospitals in the United States with four hospitals in developing countries. Results indicated that nurses and hospital administrators have similar philosophies globally regarding the importance of quality improvement initiatives.

Presently fewer than 100 hospitals have been recognized. Magnet status for excellence in nursing services rewards workplaces that place a high premium on nursing services that empower and respect nursing staff. *U.S. News & World Report* (2004) added magnet status to its criteria for judging the "Best Hospitals of 2004." Other criteria used in this hospital assessment include the mortality rate, the RN-to-patient ratio, key technologies offered, the number of discharges, patient and community services offered, and the reputation of the hospital. Magnet recognition fosters a collaborative practice and values contributions of nurses, educational support from nurses within the facility, the quality of patient care provided by institution, research-based practices, shared governance structure that encourages nursing input on decisions regarding patient care, and promotion of an empowered nursing service. Magnet hospitals boast that their nurses are more satisfied with their jobs, which they say encourages nurses to perform at peak levels. Magnet status has also been shown to be a factor in attracting physicians of the highest caliber who want to work with a highly skilled nursing staff. The Magnet Recognition Program sponsored by the American Nurses Credentialing Center is viewed by some as a catalyst for changing hospital environments. For example, one hospital wanted to focus on identifying qualities that have a positive long-term effect on nurses' job satisfaction and patient outcomes. The Magnet Recognition Program assisted this hospital in developing increased nurse clinical autonomy, more opportunity for interdisciplinary relationships, and increased availability of resources. There are multiple accounts in the literature that share how specific institutions were able to gain magnet accreditation (Johnson, Billingsley, May, Costa, & Hanson, 2004; Taylor, 2005). Aiken's studies of professional practice at magnet hospitals linked with Kanter's investigation of workplace empowerment demonstrate that these hospitals allow for more nurse empowerment (Laschinger et al., 2003).

Lewis and Matthews (1998) claim magnet hospitals "work" because they promote respect for the values, art, and science of nursing. Messmer, Jones, and Rosillo (2002) describe an example of the integration of this art and science with their institution's ongoing staff nurse research. The outcomes of the nursing staff's research conducted at this institution were identified as having great impact on the ability of the hospital to receive magnet status. Hospitals achieving magnet status are considered to be positive settings for patients, health care professionals, and the organization. (Monarch, 2003, p. 13). Trossman (2004) cites documented notable recognition for nursing services in multiple magnet institutions. DiMeglio et al. (2005) describe methods by which team building has had a positive impact on nurse satisfaction, retention, and group cohesion at their magnet hospital. They say the nurse manager's role modeling as a clinical expert, assisting with staff development, and leading the unit with outcome measurement has been instrumental in maximizing outcome success.

Another award given to hospitals reflects outcome excellence in critical care practice. It is the Beacon Award for Critical Care Excellence sponsored by the American Association of Critical Care Nurses (AACN), which recognizes the highest-quality standards in nurse recruitment, retention, and patient outcomes in critical care services. (Applications, information questions, and requirements for obtaining recognition can be obtained in either the AACN News or online at www.aacn.org.)

MENTORS AND MENTEES

It is well established that many nurses burn out and leave the profession. Raiger (2005) presents a review of the literature on burnout in nursing that offers data to support the need for mutual trust and support, vertical communication channels, and recognition of nurses. This seems to be analogous to what a mentoring culture would provide. Findings indicate that fostering trust, open communication, and respect protects nurses from burnout and facilitates a healthy work environment. More mentors need to intervene in the health care settings and transform work settings for nurses. Almada, Carafoli, Flattery, French, and McNamera (2004) and Reeves (2004) suggest several ideas that have assisted their institutions in retaining nurses by using a mentoring program. Greene and Puetzer (2002) used clinical tracking forms, planning calendars, and feedback mechanisms to increase skill and knowledge development for new nurses. Having a mentoring program helped increase retention and recruitment, as well as reinforced the need to build relationships between experienced and new nurses. Greggs-McQuilkin (2004) recommends that nursing assures a mentoring mentality. She says that the profession needs to mentor for survival since it is the interrelationships with one another that will be key to successful goal achievement for nursing. She advises nurses to focus more on collaborating and less on competing in their work settings in order to create environments in which respect, sharing, learning, and support are the standard instead of the unusual. Results from her work support that mentoring has a positive impact on retention and job satisfaction and decreases orientation costs.

Several have published their overwhelmingly positive experiences with working with preceptors, nurses, and student nurses. For example, Boswell and Wilhoit (2004) interviewed 67 new RNs regarding their perception of nurse practice quality. The nurses identified comprehensive orientation, continuing education, and mentoring as constituting high-quality practice. Papp, Markkanen, and von Bonsdorff (2003) cite findings from their study of 16 nursing students' perceptions of positive learning environments as including quality mentoring by staff nurses. Bernard (2004) describes positive outcomes regarding attitudes on aging and working with the terminally ill after students had specific role modeling with these patient populations. Certainly shadowing a role model can generate positive learning for mentees who have identified specific types of activities they are interested in observing. Mentees who are assigned a mentor or preceptor without delineating a specific purpose for the experience will likely not achieve their goals. Dunn, Ehrich, Mylonas, and Hansford (2000) conducted a phenomenological study of 25 teacher and 14 nurse students in their final semester field experience of their baccalaureate program who had been assigned a preceptor. The purpose of the research was to determine the participants' perceptions of the experience and the outcomes generated from the preceptorship:

- Role integration. Students felt they were deemed competent by a contributing member of the organization, their preceptor.
- Increased confidence. Students confirmed their self-efficacy and refocused their commitment to the profession due to their improved self-concept after working with a mentor.
- Altruism. Students felt they made a difference in their patients' or learners' lives.

Students shared multiple interactions they had been a part of with their mentor as the "most influential" aspect of the preceptorship.

Pinkerton (2003) described an 18-month mentoring program used in her institution to increase retention of RNs. Mentors cited they felt empowered and related a higher job satisfaction having experienced mentoring a new nurse. Mentees felt they gained increased self-confidence, optimism about the future, and increased critical thinking skills. This program was responsible for a 3% decrease in turnover in its first 18 months of inception. Myrick (2002) also found that "preceptors were more likely to assist with fostering critical thinking indirectly through their role modeling, facilitating, guiding, and prioritizing than they were to directly impact preceptees' critical thinking ability through questioning" (p. 161). This finding is significant because it validates the importance of having new nurses and students experience shadowing or observing proficient or expert nurses during their orientation. Experiential learning or working with a preceptor in everyday practice can assist students in appreciating how theory and research findings direct practice (Tanner, 1999; Welch, Jeffries, Lyon, Boland, & Backer, 2001). This is a significant outcome of precepting and mentoring. Aviram, Ophir, and Raviv (1998) describe how coaching and precepting students and new employees enhanced communication skills, increased cognitive and psychomotor improvement scores, increased a sense of responsibility, increased confidence, facilitated more opportunities to learn, and improved organizational, priority-setting, and interpersonal skills. Using Bandura's (1977) Social Learning Theory as a conceptual framework, they justified the use of shadowing or observational experiences with expert nurses as yielding strong learning outcomes. Nursing students learn by watching procedures performed by staff, peers, and instructors, which leads to vicarious learning. Modeling is another method of professional socialization.

According to Bandura there are two criteria for successful modeling: (1) the role model must be competent, and (2) there must be opportunities for students to practice. Then the mentee has a conscious purpose to model himself or herself after the mentor.

Partnerships between hospitals and colleges of nursing have also documented annual savings due to mentoring between faculty, staff, and students as a result of their partnerships (Novotny, Donahue, & Bhalla, 2004). Cost savings documented included less expenditure on recruitment ($79,500), employing travel nurses ($48,750), and employing adjunct faculty ($30,688). Tracy, Jagsi, Starr, and Tarbell (2004) studied the outcomes of a faculty mentoring program and found that having a role model, having increased visibility, and having someone to turn to if needed were perceived as invaluable for success by junior faculty.

FINDINGS FROM USING MENTORING EVALUATION TOOLS

Suen and Chow (2001) developed a mentoring program adapted from the English National Board (ENB) for Nursing, Midwifery, and Health Visiting to use for program evaluation of mentorships in university nursing programs in Hong Kong. Using a framework comprising the five roles of a mentor as defined by the ENB (guide, counselor, friend, assistant, and adviser), they developed an evaluation questionnaire for mentee students to use in assessing the mentors. The tool consists of 33 questions. Demographics and two subjective questions requesting their perception of the mentoring experience were also completed by the mentees. Although no validity or reliability data on this tool were given, the tool could serve as a guide for obtaining other mentees' perceptions of their preceptors or mentors. Results from this study revealed several ways to improve mentor preparation for working more effectively with students.

Hayes (1998) found a positive relationship between mentoring and student self-efficacy in her study of 238 nurse practitioner students in their final semester. She used Freeman's (1989) Mentoring Survey, which consists of 27 open- and close-ended questions eliciting the testee's perception of identifying the preceptor who was most significant in facilitating his or her career transition into the nurse practitioner role. Hayes's test-retest reliability was 0.93, with internal consistency at 0.95. Hayes also used Quality of Mentoring Tool (Caine, 1989), a 14-item Likert-type scale that also evaluates a person who was influential in the respondent's career development, the ways in which this was accomplished, and the significance of the relationship. Reliability was reported at 0.95. Significant findings were generated. Nurse practitioner students who chose their own preceptor nurse practitioner had higher scores on both instruments. The nurse practitioner students also identified the length of time they were assigned to the nurse practitioner and the preceptor's prior precepting experience. Interestingly, the areas that lowered the scores concerned indirect patient care activities or other nurse practitioner role functions such as research, consultation, case management, quality assurance, teaching, counseling, and influencing health policy. If the student had a physician assistant or physician as a preceptor, these scores were even lower. The variables that were the best predictors of mentor success were length of practicum time, with the longer the practicum the higher the mentoring score, and if the nurse practitioner preceptor had had experience being a preceptor.

Cohen (1998a, 1999, 2000) offers self-assessment instruments with interpretation and implications for mentor-employee relationships. Cohen (1998b) has also developed a video and guides for mentors and mentees. No data regarding reliability and validity are offered regarding the tools.

Noe (1988) presents a tool to measure two scales assessing career (the extent to which the mentor provided exposure and visibility, sponsorship, protection, and challenging assignments) and psychosocial (the degree to which the mentor served as a role model and provided counseling, acceptance, and confirmation) functions of mentoring with a 29-item Likert-like response. Internal consistency reliability for the career-related scale was .89 and for the psychosocial functions scale was .92. The tool seems to be applicable to measuring mentees' perceptions of their mentor functions in nursing.

CONCLUSION

After reviewing the literature, few databased articles were located that delineated outcomes of mentoring. All pointed to the need for continuing relationships between new and experienced staff, which is specifically what new mentoring models such as reverse, multiple, and co-mentoring will foster. Noe, Greenberger, and Wang (2002) suggested several strategies for future mentoring models and recommended more measurement of outcomes. For example, measurements of mentees' salary growth over their careers, promotion rates at various institutions, and number of mentees mentored in the future would be helpful. A longitudinal study that spanned 20 or 30 years of careers of nurses who had been mentored versus nurses without mentoring would be useful. Maintaining connections with all nurses will assist in expanding the mentoring culture in nursing. As Kaplan and Norton (2004) advocate, "There is no asset with greater potential for an organization than the collective knowledge possessed by all of its employees" (p. 63). Sometimes the most significant outcomes are intangible and cannot be measured with benchmark indicators. Collegiality between employees in one's work settings may well be the ultimate outcome of a mentoring culture that will facilitate more teamwork and eventual vital productivity.

REFERENCES

Aiken, L. (2005). Journey to excellence. *Reflection on Nursing Leadership, 1*, 16–19.

Aiken, L., Havens, D., & Sloane, D. (2000). The Magnet Nursing Services Recognition Program: A comparison of two groups. *American Journal of Nursing, 100,* 26–35.

Almada, P., Carafoli, K., Flattery, J., French, D., & McNamera, M. (2004). Improving the retention rate of newly graduated nurses. *Journal for Nurses in Staff Development, 20,* 268–273

American Association of Critical Care Nurses Association. (2005a). Healthy work environments. *AACN News, 22,* 2.

American Association of Critical Care Nurses. (2005b). *The AACN Standards for establishing and sustaining healthy work environments: A journey to excellence.* Aliso Viejo, CA: AACN. Retrieved October 7, 2006, from www.aacn.org.

American Nurses Association. (2004). *Scope and standards for nurse administrators.* Washington, DC: Author.

American Nurses Credentialing Center. (2003). *The Magnet recognition program health care organization application manual.* Washington, DC: Author.

Anthony, M., Standing, T., Glick, J., Duffy, M., Paschall, F., Sauer, M., et al. (2005). Leadership and nurse retention: The pivotal role of nurse managers. *Journal of Nursing Administration, 35,* 146–155.

Aviram, M., Ophir, R., & Raviv, D. (1998). Experiential learning of clinical skills by beginning nursing students: "Coaching" project by fourth year student interns. *Journal of Nursing Education, 37,* 228–231.

Bandura, A. (1977). *Social learning theory.* Englewood Cliffs, NJ: Prentice Hall.

Bernard, M. (2004). Overcoming ageism, one student at a time: Mentoring programs improve student attitudes toward older patients. *Geriatrics, 59,* 11.

Boswell, S., & Wilhoit, K. (2004). New nurses' perceptions of nursing practice and quality patient care. *Journal of Nursing Care Quality, 19,* 76–81.

Bower, F. (2000). *Nurses taking the lead: Personal qualities of effective leadership.* Philadelphia: W. B. Saunders.

Caine, R. (1989). Mentoring the novice clinical nurse specialist. *Clinical Nurse Specialist, 3,* 76–78.

Clinton, H. (2002). Respect: The not-so-secret ingredient. *American Journal of Nursing, 102,* 11.

Cohen, N. (1998a). *The principles of adult mentoring inventory.* Amherst, MA: HRD Press.

Cohen, N. (1998b). *The mentor critique form.* Amherst, MA: HRD Press.

Cohen, N. (2000). *Becoming a mentor: A video based workshop.* Amherst, MA: HRD Press.

Daloz, L. (1999). *Mentor: Guiding the journey of adult learners* (2nd ed.). San Francisco: Jossey-Bass

DiMeglio, K., Padula, C., Piatek, C., Korber, S., Barrett, A., Ducharme, M., et al. (2005). Group cohesion and nurse satisfaction: Examination of a team-building approach. *Journal of Nursing Administration, 35,* 110–120.

Dunn, S., Ehrich, L., Mylonas, A., & Hansford, B. (2000). Students' perceptions of field experience in professional development: A comparative study. *Journal of Nursing Education, 39,* 393–400.

Fields, W. L. (1991). Mentoring in nursing: A historical approach. *Nursing Outlook, 9,* 257–261.

Freeman, S. (1989). The mentor experience as perceived by nurse practitioners: Implications for curriculum design. (Doctoral dissertation, Georgia State University, 1989). *Dissertation Abstracts International, 51,* 22–44.

Gilligan, C. (1993). *In a different voice: Psychological theory and women's development* (2nd ed.). Cambridge, MA: Harvard University Press.

Goran, S. (2001). Mentorship as a teaching strategy. *Critical Care Nursing Clinics of North America, 13,* 119–129.

Greene, M., & Puetzer, M. (2002). The value of mentoring: A strategic approach to retention and recruitment. *Journal of Nursing Care Quality, 17,* 63–70.

Greggs-McQuilkin, D. (2004). Mentoring really matters: Motivate and mentor a colleague. *MEDSURG Nursing, 13,* 209, 266.

Hayes, E. (1998). Mentoring and nurse practitioner student self-efficacy. *Western Journal of Nursing Research, 20,* 521–535.

Johnson, J., Billingsley, M., May, C., Costa, L., & Hanson, K. (2004). Cause célèbre: Georgetown University Hospital's journey to magnet. *Policy, Politics, and Nursing Practice, 5,* 217–227.

Kanter, R. (1979). Power failure in management circuits. *Harvard Business Review, 57,* 65–75.

Kaplan, R., & Norton, D. (2004). Measuring the strategic readiness of intangible assets. *Harvard Business Review, 82,* 52–63, 121.

Kram, K. (1983). Phases of the mentor relationship. *Academy of Management Journal, 26,* 608–625.

Kramer, M., & Schmalenberg, C. (2003). Magnet hospital nurses describe clinical autonomy. *Nursing Outlook, 51,* 13–19.

Laschinger, H., Almost, J., & Tuer-Hodes, D. (2003). Workplace empowerment and magnet hospital characteristics. *Journal of Nursing Administration, 33,* 410–421.

Laschinger, H., Wong, C., & McMahon, L. (1999). Leader behavior impact on staff nurse empowerment, job tension, and work effectiveness. *Journal of Nursing Administration, 29,* 28–39.

Lewis, C., & Matthews, J. (1998). Magnet program designates: Exceptional nursing services. *American Journal of Nursing, 98,* 51–52.

McClure, M., & Hinshaw, A. (Eds.). (2002). *Magnet hospitals revisited: Attraction and retention of professional nurses.* Washington, DC: American Nurses Publication.

Messmer, P., Jones, S., & Rosillo, C. (2002). Using nursing research projects to meet magnet recognition program standards. *Journal of Nursing Administration, 32,* 538–543.

Monarch, K. (2003). Magnet hospitals: Powerful force for excellence. *Reflections on Nursing, 4,* 10–13.

Murray, B., Fosbinder, D., Parsons, R., Dwore, R., Dalley, K., Gustafson, G., et al. (1998). Nurse executives' leadership roles: Perceptions of incumbents and influential colleagues. *Journal of Nursing Administration, 28,* 17–24.

Myrick, F. (2002). Preceptorship and critical thinking in nursing education. *Journal of Nursing Education, 41,*154–164.

Noe, R. (1988). An investigation of the determinants of successful assigned mentoring relationships. *Personnel Psychology, 41,* 457–479.

Noe, R., Greenberger, B., & Wang, S. (2002). Mentoring: What we know and where we might go. *Research in Personnel and Human Resource Management, 21,* 124–173.

Novotny, J., Donahue, M., & Bhalla, B. (2004). The clinical partnership as strategic alliance. *Journal of Professional Nursing, 20,* 216–221.

Papp, I., Markkanen, M., & von Bonsdorff, M. (2003). Clinical environment as a learning environment: Student nurses' perceptions concerning clinical learning experiences. *Nurse Education Today, 23,* 262–268.

Pinkerton, S. (2003). Mentoring new graduates. *Nursing Economics, 21,* 202–203.

Raiger, J. (2005). Applying a cultural lens to the concept of burnout. *Journal of Transcultural Nursing, 16,* 71–76.

Reeves, K. (2004). Nurses nurturing nurses: A mentoring program. *Nurse Leader, 2,* 47–49, 53.

Roberts, A. (2000). Mentoring revisited: A phenomenological reading of the literature. *Mentoring and Tutoring, 8,* 145–170.

Shea, G. (1994). *Mentoring: Helping employees reach their own potential.* New York: American Management Association.

Shea, G. (1999). *Making the most of being mentored.* Menlo Park, CA: Crisp Learning.

Stewart, B., & Krueger, L. (1996). An evolutionary concept analysis of mentoring in nursing. *Journal of Professional Nursing, 12,* 311–321.

Suen, L., & Chow, F. (2001). Students' perceptions of the effectiveness of mentors in an undergraduate nursing program in Hong Kong. *Journal of Advanced Nursing, 36,* 505–511.

Taylor, N. (2005). The magnet pull. *Nursing Management, 36,* 36–41.

Tanner, C. (1999). Evidence-based practice: Research and critical thinking. *Journal of Nursing Education, 38,* 99.

Tracy, E., Jagsi, R., Starr, R., & Tarbell, N. (2003). Outcomes of a pilot faculty mentoring program. *American Journal of Obstetrics and Gynecology, 191,* 1846–1850.

Trossman, S. (1998). Mentoring leads to meaningful relationship, profession growth. *American Nurse, 30,* 12.

Trossman, S. (2004). Issues update: A magnetic force, ANCC program gains recognition in ensuring excellence in nursing services. *American Journal of Nursing, 104,* 68–69.

U.S. News & World Report, *Best Hospitals of 2004.* Retrieved May 2005, from http://www.com/usnews/health/hospt//tophosp.

Welch, J., Jeffries, P., Lyon, B., Boland, D., & Backer, J. (2001). Experiential learning: Integrating theory and research into practice. *Nurse Educator, 26*(5), 240–243.

CHAPTER 8

Implications for the Nursing Profession, Organizations, Mentors, and Mentees

Vance and Olson (1998) remind us that "mentoring is a privilege and an awesome responsibility" (p. 97). It is not something to take lightly, and although one of the purposes of this book is to stimulate more nurses to become part of the mentoring culture in nursing, not everyone may be able to be or may not want to be a successful mentor. They can, however, be effective at an aspect of mentoring. Just as leaders are made and not born (Bennis, 2003), nurses can be taught the skills of mentoring. They cannot be taught the art of encouraging others, however. Someone who is not self-empowered and feeling self-confident cannot encourage or lead others to become empowered. More than likely, their work setting is not conducive for encouraging others and working collaboratively. If it is a clinical setting, it is probably an extremely task-oriented and unfriendly atmosphere under the leadership of an enabling manager, or, if it is an academic setting, it is most likely a competitive, cutthroat, and uncaring environment.

Advancing a mentoring culture in nursing is necessary and timely for the profession as well as for every nurse. Every nurse can help to develop this network in the profession. There has never been a greater need for nurses to gain new skills and knowledge to empower themselves. Moreover, many health care institutions are expanding to become vast conglomerates. There are multiple systems of health care within these networks, but not all may need nurses in their workforce. That is why nurses need to be involved in the assessments for change, new planning, and decision making. They need to be connected to the right people and have the leadership skills to negotiate what is best for the nursing profession. With innovative ideas for

141

creating more effective care delivery, the escalating growth in technology, and the burgeoning costs of health care, it is not difficult to realize that care delivery cannot continue the way it has. Having a flourishing mentoring culture in nursing will assist the profession to grow exponentially. This chapter summarizes the implications of what a mentoring culture will do for the profession, the organizations that employ nurses, and the mentors and mentees.

IMPLICATIONS FOR THE NURSING PROFESSION

Chitty (2005) says "mentoring" is often the answer when successful nurses are asked: "What has been most helpful to you in your process of becoming a successful clinician, educator, or researcher?" One may wonder, "How come I did not get connected to someone who could help me with my career when I was in school? How come I am still doing the same thing and getting nowhere fast?" and "Where was the mentoring connection for me?" If graduate school was not part of a nurse's career path, probably he or she missed out on the most frequent connection to mentors. But what about connecting with others in professional organizations, colleagues at work, or college friends? What about keeping in touch with one of the professors from school? What about going to graduate school now? Perhaps none of these options is feasible now, so why not start a connection at work? How about talking with the clinical instructor who teaches nursing students on the unit? Another idea is to collaborate with some of the affiliating colleges of nursing. Maybe there is an opportunity to get involved with teaching in the college skills laboratory, tutoring students, or making a presentation at the Student Nurses Association that will lead to becoming part of a mentoring network.

Some nurses are caring for their families and parents, are very involved with their children's school organizations, or have multiple other responsibilities that do not allow time for anything else in their day. This is where a new way of thinking needs to begin that will allow the staff nurse a specific amount of time at work each shift to work on a topic, an intervention, a patient type, or some area that interests the nurse to research. (Sometimes this time may not be available depending on the staffing and acuity.) Moreover, there will need to be more delegation, more use of a team care approach, and a generally different way of thinking that every task needs the nurse involved. From this initial work, it will be possible to develop ideas to explore further the specific topic a nurse is interested in researching. The nurse will develop a better understanding of this topic and can share with others at work, through a satellite outpatient program of the health care affiliation, at a college of nursing, on a Web site, or in a journal article. The nurse will begin to make connections with other people interested in similar topics.

The nurse has now entered the mentor connection and can decide how much time and effort to spend in maximizing the growth of his or her project. The nurse can study everything available on the topic and implement some evidence-based practice interventions that no one else has yet documented. Perhaps the nurse will begin to do some consulting work. Or maybe the nurse will decide to change career paths. Whatever choices are made, the nurse has the power to make a difference with this expertise. Most likely the nurse will find, as Chitty (2005) stated, that along the road to new success, the nurse was given advice and guided by others and thereby connected with the mentoring culture. The nurse will become passionate about the chosen work and learn all that he or she can on the subject, but eventually will probably want to use the findings to make a difference. By making a difference, the nurse will most likely be empowered to make some other changes regarding his or her work. By role modeling to other nurses that things do not have to revolve around task lists at the bedside or doing all of the paperwork developed for every patient, the nurse can inspire and encourage other nurses to change too. Some of the current work done by RNs needs to be redistributed to the team. Patients and families can also participate on the team. In many instances, the nurse can assist the patient to empower himself or herself to change habits and try new ways of promoting health. Registered nurses can gain recognition for their new ways of leading in patient care and in this way benefit the entire nursing profession.

Today every nurse needs to be involved in a mentor network. It is now possible for more people than ever before to work together with more people on more projects from different corners of the earth and on a more equal footing. Work is being outsourced to areas in the world where skilled individuals will do the job effectively and more efficiently than if the work remained in the United States. Even radiographs are being sent out for interpretation in India, since it is considered more cost-effective to do so. These changes in health care delivery are being made every day, and most individuals are unaware. "So what?" one might ask. That is the key question because the answer is not clear. It would behoove the nursing profession to develop more connections with other disciplines and keep abreast of new technology and determine how it affects nursing care. Nurses need to visualize their work more broadly and create answers for the "So what?" questions. Keeping connected will help. In fact, having a mentor who is a non-health-care leader is recommended for executive nurse leaders participating in the Robert Wood Johnson Foundation Executive Nurse Fellows Program (O'Neil & Morjikian, 2003). Chief executive officers (CEOs), lawyers, accountants, entrepreneurs, and physicians can all network with nurses to expand networks. In *Life Supports: Three Nurses on the Front Lines*, Gordon (1997) describes the invisibility that nurses have had with the media. Chaffee (2000) suggests strategies for how nurses can become more visible and thus communicate contributions that nurses make more clearly and have a stronger impact on health care issues by using the media more effectively.

Today there are multiple settings for nurses to make a difference. Whether it is being involved in multidisciplinary projects, new trials of interventions, out-of-hospital health promotion activities, public health initiatives, media, journalism, or legislative work, there is a need for nursing input. Nurses need leadership skills as well as clinical skills to perform their work. The profession needs more research to identify how nurse leaders affect client outcomes, the delivery of care, and organizational change (Vance & Larson, 2002). The strongest mentoring appears to be occurring in academia with nursing doctoral students and new faculty employed at research institutions. Outcome studies are necessary to validate that obtaining federal funding, promotion and tenure, and overall career success are directly correlated with the use of mentoring structures found in some academic settings. Success with strengthening the science of nursing is directly related to the productivity of these nurse scientists. However, having a mentoring culture that involves the majority of nurses—those who practice and work with patients on a regular basis—will be most advantageous for the profession since every nurse can add to the state of the science with findings from his or her everyday practice.

IMPLICATIONS FOR ORGANIZATIONS

Satterly (2003) writes that many staff nurses feel overwhelmed and unsafe in their clinical settings and are moving out of the acute care arena to other health care facilities or even out of nursing. Her book, *Where Have All the Nurses Gone?* explains how nurses are under siege and stressed with the declining quality of care that is generally being given in the United States. Many nurses at the bedside feel they are operating without enough support from their administration. Problems include not enough professional staff, poorly prepared nurses to care for higher-acuity patients, not enough properly trained ancillary workers, and lack of resources for implementing best practice care. Organizations have learned that in order to retain experienced nurses and recruit new nurses, well-developed, planned preceptorships are mandatory. Accounts in the literature such as that by Briggs, Merk, and Mitchell (2000) describe a partnering preceptorship between several agencies in order to accomplish their vision of promoting health in central Indiana. Multiple articles detail the organization's gain in retention of nurses, lower nurse attrition rates, and improved morale when good precepting and mentoring are offered.

Chapter 4 in this book details how to set up preceptorships in health care agencies, mentoring relationships in academia, and other supportive mentoring models for graduate and undergraduate education. Organizations are beginning to develop more supportive programs for nurses with specialty training, advanced programs for specialty units, and day-long workshops for nurses in a variety of areas such as legal, ethical, caring for the dying, documentation, new technology, and a myriad of interventions. Some institutions are offering leadership workshops as well. Conflict management and negotiation strategy workshops are helpful skills for all nurse leaders (Kriteck, 2000). Mentoring will enhance mentees' knowledge of the health care system, increase their confidence and scope of thinking, and develop their communication and collaboration skills.

With more partnerships forming between academia and clinical settings, more educational programs are planned for staff. For example, nurses in critical care and the emergency department could use advice on how other hospitals have developed emergency preparedness protocols. This knowledge base has become essential for critical care nursing (Cortes, 2003). Collaboration with nursing staff from various health care agencies, professional organizations, and other disciplines will help in developing excellent educational programs. Faculty and staff can collaborate on developing programs for staff and students. There is a need to measure outcomes regarding the effect these programs are having on patient care, morale, and retention.

Organizations that sponsor any type of mentoring process will gain. They also need to reach out to staff who have been "out-networked" but still come to work and operate on their own terms, which can pose a problem for others who are complying with unit or organizational policies. An empowered manager can offer a realistic plan to assist the individual to get back into the network; an individual who did not adhere to the plan would be terminated. Keeping employees who blatantly buck the system and get away with it is not tolerable. Organizations need to support their administrators in dealing with personnel problems. If these types of problems are dealt with, they are less likely to crop up again and will reinforce the importance of every nurse adhering to organizational policies. A mentoring culture that encourages nurses to grow should flourish in settings where nurses are respected and recognized for their good work.

Fabre (2005) suggests several techniques to assist in decreasing patient errors and nurse turnover in her book, *Smart Nursing: How to Create a Positive Work Environment That Empowers and Retains Nurses*. The author promotes six management practices to assist nurses in dealing with the chaos in health care:

1. Respect
2. Simplicity
3. Flexibility
4. Integrity
5. Communication
6. Professional culture

Each of these practices (except simplicity) is fostered by a mentoring culture and has been referred to in some manner already in this book. The concept of simplicity is something for nurses to review. All of us should try to think more simply when we organize our work to accomplish goals. Perhaps instead of developing lists of tasks for people we delegate to, we should empower them to fulfill the job in whatever way they think is best. And instead of worrying about being sure to create the perfect team or join the right network, we should realize that if we are open to encouraging others, the groups will form naturally (Wheatley & Kellner-Rogers, 1996).

Cleary and Rice (2005) look at collaboration between schools of nursing, state government, and health care institutions in strategizing ways to manage the nursing shortage. There are multiple initiatives that staff nurses need to be involved in so that the nursing workforce is developed most prudently.

IMPLICATIONS FOR MENTORS AND MENTEES

The reason every nurse needs a mentor is that each nurse is different and a recipe or a one-size-fits-all mentality is not going to be effective. Joel and Kelly (2002) suggest there is a special need for mentoring models for preparing nurse leaders, developing minority nurses, and preparing nurse scholars. One model of international mentoring is offered through the Chiron Mentor-Fellow Program sponsored by Sigma Theta Tau International (STTI) and promises to "advance nursing and the mentee's career." STTI offers members the opportunity to work with mentors and develop leadership skills in a formalized fellowship through Chiron: The Mentor-Fellow Forum. During a 12-month program, nurses who desire skill development in specific leadership areas are guided by experienced mentors as they implement individualized plans and participate in group activities. Potential mentors and fellows are encouraged to seek out partners and apply as a pair to the program.

Just about every nursing professional organization newsletter or journal cites how critical it is for nurses to mentor others. For example, the American Association of Critical Care Nurses has a picture of senior nursing students on the brochure advertising the National Teaching Institute Critical Care Exposition. The brochure also notes that "it is critical for experienced and veteran nurses to welcome students, along with other young nurses and those in training into the American Association of Critical Care Nursing's family."

Once again the concept of mentoring may be used too freely, and what the STTI is really sponsoring is a year of coaching, not mentoring. It will depend on the mentor and mentee as to just what transpires. However, coaching a mentee to conduct research, present findings, and publish in a refereed journal; or develop an evidence-based practice protocol and disseminate its use; or apply for funding for a project is assisting someone to increase his or her leadership skills. Similarly, mentors in academia can guide a student with his or her research over one semester, connect the student to a funded researcher in the mentee's field, or advise by means of e-mail during a sabbatical and still have mentored or coached them. Many nurses have connected with mentors over the Internet and communicate through e-mail. This is just another way of obtaining advice, and it is beneficial to have someone outside one's own institution or even one's field (Whiting & de Janesz, 2004). The idea of the classic long-term dyad relationship is not the only type of mentoring there is, and more and more nurses will be accessing multiple mentors across their careers.

Wickman and Sjodin (1996) describe how mentoring influences people and provides strategies for both the mentor and mentee in generating additional professional growth and development. In fact, this serves to validate that mentoring is a time-honored tradition and an important catalyst for people in achieving success in personal, professional, economic, and emotional areas.

For example, beginning staff nurses need seasoned, experienced preceptors to guide them through the maze of nursing in order to achieve competency. It will be more up to a peer mentoring network for nurses to proceed to proficiency and, for nurses who are very fortunate, expert status.

Benner's (1984; Benner, Tanner, & Chesla, 1996) Acquisition of Skills Model is important for both mentors and mentees to review since it clearly identifies behaviors at each level of nursing expertise. It is only by having a standard by which to measure one's competency that the mentee can progress and accomplish his or her goals.

Mentoring is defined as any supportive relationship in which the individual or mentee receives guidance and encouragement. Often this guidance is reciprocal, that is, it is given back and forth between mentor and mentee. Peer or co-mentoring is a phenomenon that has caught on with the great majority of 20- and 30-year-olds. The guidance or coaching from peers can occur with a variety of learning opportunities: practicing and mastering clinical skills, tutoring for the National Council Licensure Examination (NCLEX) or a certification exam, offering strategies for succeeding with conflicts and departmental problems, offering troubleshooting advice for technology adjustments, obtaining federal funding for research, career planning, editing manuscripts, connecting individuals to networks, and legal or ethical advice, among many others. Other opportunities that mentors can help others with refer to providing experience to practice a specific skill—leadership, management, or clinical skills, for example. Mentors can also role-model for mentees how to deal with particularly tough negotiations, policy development strategizing, and multiple challenging situations. Mentors also have a responsibility to instill pride in mentees and to role-model for them that pride matters more than money (Katzenbach, 2000, 2003).

CONCLUSION

Periodically it is beneficial to review the various mentors one has had. Not everyone will have a legendary mentor. There is a tendency to have mentors when one makes a change in career or during shifts from one developmental stage to another in one's professional growth. Hopefully, people can identify their mentoring connections and realize that, in most instances, these connections helped them achieve goals. But there are always some who are too arrogant to think they ever had a mentor and feel they achieved their career accomplishments solely by themselves. They do not realize the power of a team and often prefer to work in isolation. It is essential that these nurses realize what Kaplan and Norton (2004) believe: "No asset has greater potential for an organization than the collective knowledge possessed by all of its employees" (p. 63).

Most frequently a mentor empowers an individual in some unique way to accomplish goals. Having self-esteem will allow the mentee to recognize others for their assistance. It seems that the more mentors one has, the more of one's potential is actualized, and the more accomplishments one experiences. It is probably correct to assume that the number of positive mentoring encounters far exceeds the small number of negative ones. How fortunate for those who can visualize having had a mentoring connection that included encouragement, challenges, constructive feedback, role modeling, and, for the mentor "to [be able to] fall back willingly to allow the mentee to walk beyond" (Schwiebert, 2000, p. 169). Even being able to give one or two of these gifts to another will facilitate the mentoring culture in nursing. If the mentoring culture is to take root, it is important that every individual, not just the academics, strive to fulfill more global goals in order to benefit the profession.

REFERENCES

Benner, P. (1984). *From novice to expert: Excellence and power in clinical nursing practice*. Menlo Park, CA: Addison-Wesley.

Benner, P., Tanner, C., & Chesla, C. (1996). *Expertise in nursing practice: Caring, clinical judgment, and ethics*. New York: Springer Publishing.

Bennis, W. (2003). *On becoming a leader: Leadership classic—updated and expanded* (2nd ed.). Reading, MA: Addison-Wesley.

Briggs, L., Merk, S., & Mitchell, B. (2000). *Collaboration for the promotion of nursing: Building partnerships for the future*. Indianapolis, IN: Sigma Theta Tau International.

Chaffee, M. (2000). Health communications: Nursing education for increased visibility and effectiveness. *Journal of Professional Nursing, 16,* 31–38.

Chitty, K. (2005). *Professional nursing: Concepts and challenges* (4th ed.). St. Louis: Elsevier Saunders.

Cleary, B., & Rice, R. (Eds.). (2005). *Nursing workforce development: Strategic state initiatives*. New York: Springer Publishing.

Cortes, T. (2003). Developing passion and excellence in critical care nursing: Proposed solutions to current challenges in critical care. *Policy, Politics, and Nursing Practice, 5,* 21–24.

Fabre, J. (2005). *Smart nursing: How to create a positive work environment that empowers and retains nurses*. New York: Springer Publishing.

Gordon, S. (1997). *Life support: Three nurses on the front lines*. Boston: Little, Brown.

Joel, L., & Kelly, L. (2002). *The nursing experience: Trends, challenges, and transitions* (4th ed.). New York: McGraw-Hill.

Kaplan, R., & Norton, D. (2004). Measuring the strategic readiness of intangible assets. *Harvard Business Review, 82,* 52–63, 121.

Katzenbach, J. (2000). *Peak performance: Aligning the hearts and minds of your employees*. Boston: Harvard Business School Press.

Katzenbach, J. (2003). *Why pride matters more than money: The power of the world's greatest motivational force.* New York: Crown.

Kriteck, P. (2000). *Negotiating at an uneven table: A practical approach to working with difference and diversity.* San Francisco: Jossey-Bass.

O'Neil, E., & Morjikian, R. (2003). Nursing leadership: Challenges and opportunities. *Policy, Politics, and Nursing Practice, 4,* 173–179.

Satterly, F. (2003). *Where have all the nurses gone?* Amherst, NY: Prometheus.

Schwiebert, V. (2000). *Mentoring: Creating connected, empowered relationships.* Alexandria, VA: American Counseling Association.

Vance, C., & Larson, E. (2002). Leadership research in business and health care. *Journal of Nursing Scholarship, 34,* 165–171.

Vance, C., & Olson, R. (Eds.). (1998). *The mentor connection in nursing.* New York: Springer Publishing.

Wheatley, M., & Kellner-Rogers, M. (1996). *A simpler way.* San Francisco: Berrett-Koehler.

Whiting, V., & de Janesz, S. (2004). Mentoring in the 21st century: Using the Internet to build skills and networks. *Journal of Management Education, 28,* 275–294.

Wickman, F., & Sjodin, T. (1996). *Mentoring: The most obvious yet overlooked key to achieving more in life than you ever dreamed possible.* New York: McGraw-Hill.

Index